O A P L

OXFORD AMERICAN PAIN LIBRARY

Migraine and Headache

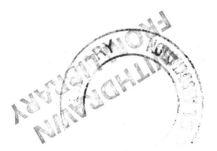

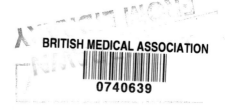

O A P L
OXFORD AMERICAN PAIN LIBRARY

Migraine and Headache

2nd Edition

Alexander Mauskop, MD, FAAN

Director, New York Headache Center
Professor of Clinical Neurology
State University of New York
Downstate Medical Center

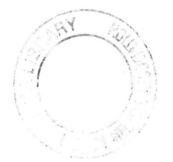

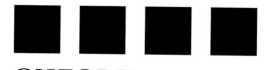

OXFORD
UNIVERSITY PRESS

OXFORD

UNIVERSITY PRESS

Oxford University Press is a department of the University of Oxford.
It furthers the University's objective of excellence in research, scholarship,
and education by publishing worldwide.

Oxford   New York
Auckland   Cape Town   Dar es Salaam   Hong Kong   Karachi
Kuala Lumpur   Madrid   Melbourne   Mexico City   Nairobi
New Delhi   Shanghai   Taipei   Toronto

With offices in
Argentina   Austria   Brazil   Chile   Czech Republic   France   Greece
Guatemala   Hungary   Italy   Japan   Poland   Portugal   Singapore
South Korea   Switzerland   Thailand   Turkey   Ukraine   Vietnam

Oxford is a registered trademark of Oxford University Press in the UK
and certain other countries.

Published in the United States of America by
Oxford University Press
198 Madison Avenue, New York, NY 10016

© Oxford University Press 2013

Library of Congress Cataloging-in-Publication Data

Mauskop, Alexander.
Migraine and headache / Alexander Mauskop. -- 2nd ed.
p. ; cm. — (Oxford American pain library)
Includes bibliographical references.
ISBN 978-0-19-986204-7 (pbk. : alk. paper)
I. Title.   II. Series: Oxford American pain library.
[DNLM: 1. Migraine Disorders.   2. Headache. WL 344]
616.8'4912—dc23   2012016024

9 8 7 6 5 4 3 2 1
Printed in the United States of America
on acid-free paper

Disclosures

Dr. Mauskop has served on the advisory boards, conducted research, or given promotional lectures on behalf of the following companies whose products are discussed in the book: Allergan, Abbott Laboratories, Bristol-Myers Squibb, Endo, GlaxoSmithKline, Johnson and Johnson, Merck, Novartis, Pfizer, and Zogenix. He is the owner of Migralex, Inc.

>

Dedication

For my parents, Toba and Marton Mauskop, who survived Auschwitz, outlived the Soviet Union, and preserved their faith, sanity, and dignity.

Acknowledgment

I thank my dedicated colleagues at the New York Headache Center, and particularly Dr. Christina Sun-Edelstein, for help with this manuscript.

Contents

Introduction

Approximately 30 million Americans are afflicted with migraine headaches or chronic migraines which have a detrimental effect on the quality of life of many sufferers.[1] Glen Solomon and colleagues[2] used detailed questionnaires to document the impact of migraine disorders. Among other common head pain disorders are tension headaches, which occur in up to 80% of the population, and are usually too mild to lead to a doctor visit, unless they become chronic. Most patients seeking medical attention for head pain have one of these two types of headaches. Nevertheless, less than half of the 30 million migraine sufferers see a physician and learn their diagnosis. The majority do not realize that they have migraine headaches. Many patients classify migraines as sinus headaches or what some patients unfortunately call "normal headaches." Other relatively less common headache disorders include cluster headaches, which can be severe and devastating, and brain tumor headaches, which are usually easy to diagnose as they are accompanied by other neurological symptoms. Aneurysm related headache is a common concern among patients, but an aneurysm typically causes a single catastrophic headache as opposed to repeated episodes as in other headache syndromes.

The incidence of migraine in general population is about 12% but waiting room surveys indicate that as many as one third of patients in doctors' offices suffer from migraines. This difference is probably accounted for by comorbidities such as irritable bowel syndrome, depression, anxiety and obesity—conditions that are more likely to bring the patient into the office. A staggering 4% of the population suffers from headaches almost daily.[3] A common question patients have is whether their doctor has ever seen someone with a headache that lasted two years. Unfortunately, the majority of patients visiting headache clinics have chronic headaches. While women suffer from migraines three times more often than men, they constitute 90% of patients who seek help for their headaches. Women tend to seek help for their medical problems more readily than men do; however, even women often don't mention headaches to their primary care doctors or only mention them as an afterthought. One explanation is the persistent prejudices that can make women think that headache is not a serious disorder, but rather a weakness of character or something that only affects neurotic women.

James Lance in the introduction to the first edition of his now classic textbook on headaches published in 1969 describes the attitude of family members, friends and co-workers, as well as of many physicians: "It is easy for a person who has never been troubled with headaches to lose patience with those who are plagued by them. The reaction of the virtuous observer may pass through a phase of sympathetic concern to one of frustrated tolerance and, finally, to a mood of irritation and resentment in which the recurrence of headaches is attributed to a defective personality or escape from unpleasant life situations."[4]

Hang up a sign in your waiting room: "Please mention to the doctor if you suffer from headaches" and you will see how many patients will come forward. And if you think this will increase your burden, well it might, but you will also significantly improve your patients' lives and your job satisfaction. There is no better reward than to hear: "Doctor, you've changed my life," It is remarkable how far we have advanced in the treatment of headaches in the past 15 years— the resources we now have at our disposal relieve the suffering of the majority of headache sufferers. New treatments are being developed and several may become available in the next few years, further improving the lives of these patients.

References

1. Lipton RB, Bigal ME, Diamond M et al. Migraine prevalence, disease burden, and the need for preventive therapy. *Neurolog.y* 2007; 68:343–349.

2. Solomon GD, Skobieranda FG, Gragg LA. Does quality of life differ among headache diagnoses? Analysis using the medical outcomes study instrument. *Headache* 1994; 34(3):143–147.

3. Scher AI, Stewart WF, Liberman J, Lipton RB. Prevalence of frequent headache in a population sample. *Headache.* 1998;38(7):497–506.

4. Lance J, Goadsby PJ. *Mechanism and Management of Headache.* Butterworth-Heinemann; 7 edition, November 26, 2004.

Chapter 1

Classification and Diagnosis of Primary Headaches

Migraine

The International Headache Society's (IHS) highly detailed classification of headaches (see ihs-classification.org), now in its second edition, has become an important research tool, albeit with modest practical applications.[1] Danish physician Jes Olesen was the major force behind this effort. Migraine diagnosis is based on the description of symptoms reported by patients. The most common type of migraine is migraine without aura, and its features include moderate or severe pain, unilateral location, throbbing quality of pain, worsening with light physical activity, sensitivity to light and noise, and nausea or vomiting. All or any particular set of features need not be present. For example, bilateral nonthrobbing pain that is severe and made worse by light physical activity and is accompanied by photophobia and phonophobia is classified as migraine. A patient who has mild unilateral pain that is throbbing and is accompanied by nausea also suffers from migraine. Some patients will not report sensitivity to light or noise, but when asked, they will admit that they prefer being in a darkened and quiet environment. Many also become very sensitive to odors and touch. According to a recent report,[2] a simplified way to screen for migraines with a high degree of accuracy is to ask your patients three questions:

1. In the past three months, has the headache stopped you from doing something you wanted to do or, in other words, was the headache in any way disabling for at least one day?
2. In the past three months, has the headache made you feel nauseated or sick to your stomach?
3. In the past three months, has the headache made you feel sensitive to light?

These three features were found to be the most predictive of migraine diagnosis, and if two of these are present, it is very likely that the patient is suffering from migraines.

At times, we diagnose migraine in patients who do not quite fulfill all of the required criteria. The official IHS classification categorizes this condition as probable migraine—between 10% and 40% of patients fall into this category. The treatment approach to probable migraine is similar to the treatment of definite migraine.

Migraine aura is present in up to one third of patients with migraines,[3] and for those patients, the official diagnosis is migraine with aura. Aura typically consists of scintillations (flashing zigzags, flickering lights, and the like) with or without complete obscuration of vision, which usually progresses from the periphery to the midline. It usually occurs in the same half of each eye (homonymous hemianopia), which patients often misinterpret as occurring in one eye only. Some patients have only loss of vision without any positive visual phenomena or have narrowing of the visual field to the point of having tunnel vision. Aura lasts anywhere from five to 60 minutes, but most commonly it lasts 20 to 30 minutes. Rarely, aura symptoms persist for hours, days, and months, often causing disability (classified as persistent aura without infarction). Some patients have only auras without headaches (typical aura without headache), or both aura without headache and typical migraine headache without aura. In addition to visual aura, sensory symptoms may follow the visual symptoms and also usually last five to 60 minutes. Numbness or paresthesias usually spread from the hand up the arm or skip the arm and move up to involve half of the face, at times including the tongue. Some patients with sensory aura may also feel weak in the same extremity, but it is mild weakness or often just awkwardness due to sensory impairment. This should not be mistaken for hemiparesis. In some patients, aura consists of aphasia—difficulty finding words or difficulty thinking and speaking clearly. Frequent attacks of visual aura can become disabling even in the absence of a severe headache and can cause severe anticipatory anxiety.

Menstrual migraines are almost never preceded by an aura. Approximately 60% of women with migraines report having attacks around the time of their menstruation and 14% have attacks only with their periods. Postpartum headaches can result from a variety of causes, such as epidural anesthesia complicated by a dural puncture. Cerebral venous thrombosis, eclampsia, and stroke are among the more serious conditions. If headache develops weeks after delivery, common causes and triggers include hypothyroidism, sleep deprivation, stress, and hormonal changes.

Hemiplegic Migraine

When significant weakness is present and persists into the headache phase of migraine, this is termed hemiplegic migraine. This disorder can be hereditary or idiopathic. There is a practical need for differentiating sensory aura with some perceived weakness from true hemiplegic migraine, as triptans are contraindicated in patients with hemiplegic migraines but not in patients who have migraine with aura. However, this contraindication does not stem from a scientific study or clinical experience, but was put in place based on speculation that because triptans cause some cerebral vasoconstriction and the aura symptoms are also due to vasoconstriction, triptans could provoke a stroke. In fact, aura symptoms are primarily due to the inhibition of neuronal activity and not to vasoconstriction. Several headache experts reported the safe use of triptans in patients with hemiplegic and basilar migraine.[4,5] However, as a general rule, patients with hemiplegia should not be prescribed triptans and should be evaluated by a neurologist.

Basilar-Type Migraine

Also known as Bickerstaff migraine, basilar-type migraine received its name because symptoms of this condition can also occur with ischemia in the distribution of basilar artery. These symptoms include dizziness or vertigo, tinnitus, diplopia, dysarthria, and bilateral peripheral dysesthesias followed by an occipital headache. A large epidemiological study performed in Denmark discovered that patients diagnosed as having basilar migraine in fact suffer from migraine with aura.[6] It is likely that this diagnosis will be removed from the next edition of classification of headaches. The importance of this change is that triptans are contraindicated in patients with basilar migraine, so doctors treating patients with diplopia, vertigo, and other symptoms attributed to basilar migraine will be able to prescribe these medications without fear of serious side effects or legal action.

Chronic Migraine

Chronic migraine is surprisingly common. According to three epidemiological studies conducted in three different countries, 1 to 5% of the population has headaches on more than 15 days each month.[3] The existence of chronic migraines at first was denied, then debated, and finally accepted; its definition was debated, accepted, revised, and still continues to be debated. Simply put, if headaches occur on more than 15 days a month and if on some days migraine features are present, then the diagnosis is chronic migraine. The current definition requires the presence of migrainous features on at least eight days, but in practice there is no need to stick to this specific number. There is indirect evidence to suggest that the presence of only a few migraine attacks a month indicates a migrainous character of chronic headache and it should be treated as such. Published data suggests that even in patients who suffer from fewer than six migraines a month along with tension-type headaches, both types of headaches respond well to sumatriptan, suggesting that migrainous process is responsible for both types of headaches. Sumatriptan does not relieve tension-type headaches if the patient does not suffer from migraines as well.

Triptans are highly effective for the treatment of migraine headaches, but when a headache responds to a triptan, it does not mean that the headache is necessarily a migraine. Headaches caused by subarachnoid hemorrhage due to a ruptured aneurysm and headaches due to a brain tumor can also respond to triptans. The converse is also true—lack of response to a triptan does not mean that the headache is not a migraine.

Migraine Status

This refers to a migraine attack that has lasted for longer than 72 hours with pain that has remained severe. If the pain is mild, the diagnosis is probable migraine without aura.

Migrainous Infarction

This is a rare condition and is usually manifested by persistence of aura symptoms with an infarction documented on a computed tomography scan or magnetic resonance image. It tends to occur in patients who suffer from migraine with aura and have other risk factors for strokes. In young women who constitute the majority of migraine sufferers, common risk factors include estrogen-containing contraceptives and smoking.

Tension-Type Headache

Often defined as nonmigraines, they are mild or moderate in intensity, nonpulsatile in quality, bilateral in location, not made worse by light physical activity, and not accompanied by nausea, photophobia, or phonophobia. Some patients have tenderness of pericranial muscles and some do not. Chronic tension-type headache is present when the headache occurs on more than 15 days each month.

Cluster Headache

These headaches are often so extremely intense that they lead to thoughts of suicide. There are about five times as many men with cluster headaches as women and many more smokers than in the general population (although quitting smoking does not seem to stop the headaches).[7] Bouts of cluster headaches typically last one to three months and occur once or twice a year, but they can skip a year or several years. Interestingly, cluster headache patients tend to cluster throughout the year—many appear to develop their cluster periods in the same month or two, but this clustering occurs in different months each year. It is not clear what environmental factors may play a role, but anecdotally the author observed that increased solar activity may be a trigger. In 10 to 15% of patients, cluster headaches change from episodic form to chronic form or start as chronic and occur daily for years. During cluster episodes, attacks occur once or several times a day, often at night, and usually wake the patient from sleep at the same time every night. The duration of attacks is 30 to 90 minutes, but they can last for up to three hours. Characteristic features include piercing pain, ipsilateral lacrimation and nasal congestion with watery discharge, forehead and facial sweating, miosis, ptosis, and eyelid edema. Complaints of nasal congestion and runny nose can lead to an erroneous diagnosis of sinus headaches. Unilateral pain is sometimes misinterpreted as that of a migraine. The salient feature of cluster headaches that helps differentiate them from migraines, besides lacrimation and nasal discharge, is agitation. Most migraine patients prefer to stay motionless, while cluster sufferers cannot stay still and typically rock, pace, moan, and hit their head with a fist or against the wall. At times patients report having ipsilateral occipital pain or tenderness and that pressing in that area provides temporary relief. Physical examination during an attack may reveal Horner's syndrome and conjunctival injection. Many cluster headache sufferers have a ruddy face with thick skin and deep furrows.

Paroxysmal Hemicrania

This condition can be both episodic and chronic, and it is also called indomethacin-sensitive headache because of its dramatic response to indomethacin. The clinical features are very similar to those of cluster headaches with unilateral pain, nasal congestion, and lacrimation. However, the attacks usually last two to five and up to 30 minutes and occur much more often—five to 30 times daily. Women are more often afflicted by this condition than are men.

Hemicrania Continua

This is another strictly unilateral and indomethacin-sensitive headache that is present daily and continuously without pain-free periods. It tends to be moderate in intensity with periods of severe pain with few associated autonomic symptoms. This headache is often misdiagnosed as chronic migraine or chronic tension-type headache, which delays proper treatment with indomethacin.

Medication-Overuse Headache

This headache has also been described as rebound headache and was first observed in workers at a pharmaceutical company in Switzerland who were given free samples of an analgesic phenacetin and developed daily headaches. Researchers reported a similar phenomenon caused by ergots in a 1951 study. Opioid analgesics and a short-acting barbiturate, butalbital, are suspected to also cause medication overuse headache, based on a one-year long study of headache progression by Marcelo Bigal and his colleagues.[8] This type of headache supposedly results from ongoing withdrawal from the medication that is being overused. Caffeine is the only substance proved to cause withdrawal headache in a double-blind trial.[9] We do see many patients who improve after stopping daily intake of triptans, nonsteroidal anti-inflammatory drugs, and other analgesics, but this could be due to a variety of factors, including lifestyle changes or other interventions (prophylactic medications, supplements, botulinum toxin injections), or in part due to the therapeutic power of the encounter with a physician. While many patients improve after stopping daily abortive drugs, a fair number has to return to taking daily triptans or NSAIDs in order to control their headaches and remain functional. Patients who succeed on this regimen of daily triptans or NSAIDs typically remain on a steady amount of medication for long periods of time without the need to escalate the dose and without loss of efficacy. It is rare, but has been encountered by the author, that a patient with daily headaches can remain on a steady daily dose of butalbital/caffeine combination or an opioid analgesic for many years with good relief, no side effects, normal functioning, and without developing tolerance (i.e., the need to escalate the dose over time).

Hypnic Headache

First described by Neil Raskin,[10] this headache syndrome typically occurs in the elderly and wakes them from sleep. The headache is usually diffuse, not very severe, lasts 15 to 180 minutes, and occurs every night. Nightly doses of caffeine and lithium have been found to be effective in preventing these headaches.

Cervicogenic Headache

These headaches are caused by a disorder of nerves, muscles, ligaments, and bones of the neck. A recent report indicates that not only upper neck structures but even disc disease in the lower cervical spine can cause headaches.[11] The pain of cervicogenic headache is not always occipital, but it can also radiate to the frontal region, in the distribution of the first branch of the trigeminal nerve. These headaches are more common in the elderly and are characterized by neck muscle spasm. They are often accompanied by limited range of movements. Cervicogenic headaches are often worse upon awakening, possibly due to awkward positions that patients may end up in while asleep. Examination is remarkable for neck muscle spasm and limitation in the range of movements.

Patients with rheumatoid arthritis who develop a new headache must be evaluated for the presence of atlantoaxial joint disease, which carries the risk of spinal cord injury. This is accomplished by flexion and extension x-ray or computed tomography scan views of the cervical spine.

Another condition that should be considered in the differential diagnosis is internal carotid or vertebral artery dissection, which can present with a unilateral headache and neck pain. Dissection can occur after a trauma to the neck, whiplash injury, or chiropractic manipulation or at times without an obvious cause. Only 15% of patients have pain in the head and neck without any neurological symptoms. Most patients with dissection develop neurological deficits. Horner's syndrome occurs in some patients with carotid artery dissection, which can confuse the diagnosis of dissection with cluster headache. Vertebral artery dissection often results in a stroke. Magnetic resonance angiography is usually diagnostic, but in some patients with vertebral artery dissection conventional angiography is necessary.

Spasm of neck muscles is frequently present in patients with migraines. This can be a splinting response to the pain of the headache, which may worsen the headache, causing a vicious cycle. In some patients, neck pain with muscle spasm can be the initiating trigger. These headaches are still classified as migraine and not cervicogenic headaches if typical migraine features are present.

Primary Headache Associated with Sexual Activity

This headache is divided into preorgasmic and orgasmic headaches. Preorgasmic headache is usually characterized by a dull ache in the head, neck, and at times jaw muscles. Orgasmic headache is typically explosive and severe and lasts from minutes to hours. The first occurrence of orgasmic headache needs to be investigated urgently as it could be due to a rupture of an intracranial aneurysm or arterial dissection.

Primary Stabbing Headache (Icepick Pains)

Approximately 40% of migraine patients experience this type of headache, which has also been called jabs and jolts syndrome, in addition to their migraines.[12] Patients are often concerned about the underlying cause of this pain, but the condition is benign, albeit of unknown etiology. The pain is usually sharp and very brief, lasting a few seconds, and in most patients it occurs in various locations. The pain intensity is much less severe than the pain of trigeminal neuralgia and is not of electric-like quality that is typical of neuralgia. The pain distribution, however, is in the first branch of the trigeminal nerve—frontal, temporal, and parietal areas. The frequency of these stabs varies from several in a year to many each day.

Exploding Head Syndrome

This condition is not really a headache because the patient does not experience any pain, but it is often reported as a headache. It always wakes patients from sleep and they feel like an explosion went off in their head, at times with a perception of a flash of light. The sensation is momentary and patients are able to go back to sleep. Attacks tend to be infrequent and do not require treatment.

References

1. The International Classification of Headache Disorders. *Cephalalgia*. 2004;24(suppl 1).

2. Lipton RB, Dodick D, Sadovsky R, et al. A self-administered screener for migraine in primary care: The ID Migraine™ validation study. *Neurology*. 2003;61:375–382.

3. Olesen J, Goadsby PJ, Ramadan NM, Tfelt-Hansen P, Welch KMA, eds. *The Headaches*. 3rd ed. Philadelphia: Lippincott Williams and Wilkins; 2006.

4. Klapper J, Mathew N, Nett R. Triptans in the treatment of basilar migraine and migraine with prolonged aura. *Headache*. 2001;41:981–984.

5. Artto V, Nissilä M, Wessman M, Palotie A, Färkkilä M, Kallela M. Treatment of hemiplegic migraine with triptans. *Eur J Neurol*. 2007;14:1053–1056.

6. Kirchmann M, Thomsen LL, Olesen J. Basilar-type migraine: Clinical, epidemiologic, and genetic features. *Neurology*. 2006;66:880–886.

7. Ekbom K, Svensson DA, Träff H, Waldenlind E. Age at onset and sex ratio in cluster headache: Observations over three decades. *Cephalalgia.* 2002;22:94–100.

8. Bigal ME, Serrano D, Buse D, Scher A, Stewart WF, Lipton RB. Acute migraine medications and evolution from episodic to chronic migraine: A longitudinal population-based study. *Headache* 2008;48:1157–1168.

9. Silverman K, Evans SM, Strain EC, Griffiths RR. Withdrawal syndrome after the double-blind cessation of caffeine consumption. *N Engl J Med.* 1992;327:1109–1114.

10. Raskin NH. The hypnic headache syndrome. *Headache.* 1988;28:534–536.

11. Diener HC, Kaminsk M, Stappert G, Stolke D, Schoch B. Lower cervical disc prolapse may cause cervicogenic headache: Prospective study in patients undergoing surgery. *Cephalalgia.* 2007;27:1050–1054.

12. Raskin NH, Schwartz RK. Icepick-like pain. *Neurology.* 1980;30:203–205.

Chapter 2

Pathophysiology of Migraine and Other Headaches

Migraine and tension-type headaches are two distinct disorders; however, they can also be considered to belong to a spectrum of a single disease. At the ends of this spectrum, migraine and tension-type headaches are clearly different, but many patients have headaches that fall in the middle of the spectrum or have both types of headaches. As mentioned, tension-type headaches in patients who also suffer from migraines respond well to migraine-specific medications such as sumatriptan. However, triptans are ineffective in patients who have only tension-type headaches, suggesting that at the extremes of the spectrum these two conditions are indeed distinct. Certain imaging and neurophysiological studies can also differentiate typical migraine and tension-type headaches.

Because migraines cause disability in millions of patients, while tension-type headaches do not, most of the scientific research has been devoted to migraines. We know that tension-type headaches result from a combination of both peripheral (mostly muscular), as well as central brain mechanisms. Tension-type headaches lack the biochemical (serotonin, nitric oxide, magnesium, and other) and some neurophysiological (such as cortical spreading depression, central nervous system hyperexcitability, etc.) changes that accompany migraine headaches. The transformation of episodic tension-type headache into chronic, a process that also occurs with migraines, may involve the phenomenon of central sensitization. After a prolonged barrage of painful stimuli into the central nervous system, certain central neurons become hypersensitive and a cascade of neurochemical events causes the pain to become self-sustaining.

Migraine is a genetic disorder, with double of the risk of migraine in first-degree relatives of patients who suffer from migraine without aura. This risk is four times greater when aura is present. Genetic linkage studies have identified specific genes responsible for the rarely seen hemiplegic migraine, although in some families the abnormal gene was found on chromosome 19 and in others, on chromosome 1. A minor allele on chromosome 8 was found to be more prevalent in patients with migraine with and without aura. Risk of migraine with aura is increased in patients who are homozygous for C677T genotype of the methylenetetrahydrofolate reductase (MTHFR) gene. Patients homozygous for this allele have elevated homocysteine levels. It is possible that this accounts for the increased risk of strokes in patients with migraine with aura. It is clear that both migraine with and without aura are caused by multiple genetic abnormalities, accounting for such heterogeneity of the migraine phenotype. It is possible that with advances in genetic research we will be able to identify different migraine subtypes, which in turn may help predict response to various therapeutic interventions.

Genetic factors are very difficult to discern in episodic tension-type headaches because of the high prevalence of this condition; but chronic tension-type headaches are associated with a threefold increase in the risk of this condition in first-degree relatives.

Migraine is no longer considered a vascular disorder, but rather an illness originating in the brain with secondary vascular changes. The fact that many vascular conditions are accompanied by migraine headaches suggests that vascular factors also play a role, although it is possible that they just share common genetic mechanisms. The brains of migraine patients, even in the absence of recent attacks, are more excitable than the brains of people who do not suffer from migraines. They also tend to have lower levels of magnesium.[1] Migraine sufferers have low magnesium levels not only in the brain but also in the rest of their body.[2,3] Almost any person can develop a single attack of migraine given enough triggers (sleep deprivation, dehydration, alcohol, stress, etc.); however, migraine sufferers have a much lower threshold. The brainstem center where the migraine process supposedly begins has been identified by positron emission tomography and magnetic resonance imaging studies.[4] This center is thought to receive triggering input from other parts of the nervous system (hypothalamus, limbic system, cortex) and humoral factors (circulating hormones, hypomagnesemia, hypothyroidism). Once this center is activated, a cascade of neuronal and neurochemical events causes neurogenic inflammation and sensitization of trigeminal nucleus caudalis, with subsequent transmission of signals to the thalamus and cortex where pain is perceived. Dorsal raphe nucleus, locus coeruleus, periaqueductal gray, hypothalamus, and superior salivary nucleus are some of the other structures intimately involved in the migraine process.

The phenomenon of central sensitization, extensively researched by Rami Burstein and colleagues, occurs in many migraine patients.[5] Central sensitization produces allodynia or cutaneous hypersensitivity and muscle tenderness. Migraine attacks appear to respond poorly to treatment if it is given after the onset of central sensitization.

Cortical spreading depression underlies the phenomenon of visual aura and precedes the activation of the brainstem center.[6] Cortical spreading depression may be caused by calcium flux and signal propagation along the glial cells rather than by neurons, and possibly by independent signal propagation along blood vessels. Neurotransmitters involved in the migraine process include serotonin, calcitonin gene-related peptide (CGRP), nitric oxide, substance P, kinins, glutamate, and many others. Gap junction blockers, which impede cortical spreading depression by inhibiting glial cell communication, are in development for the prevention of migraines.[7] Abortive therapy with CGRP antagonists, appears to be at least as effective as with triptans.[8,9] Unlike triptans, CGRP antagonists do not carry the risk of coronary vasoconstriction.

Population studies have shown that migraine with aura is associated with an increased risk of stroke. Although the relationship appears to be stronger in younger patients, the effect may persist in older ones as well. This risk is significantly increased by smoking and the use of estrogen-containing oral contraceptives. Furthermore, there is evidence that migraine with aura is associated with an increased risk of any ischemic vascular event, including coronary artery disease. At present, the mechanisms underlying the relationship between stroke and migraine with aura are not well understood, but both neuronal and vascular dysfunction are likely to be involved. In addition to the MTHFR gene abnormality, several theories have been proposed, which include microcirculatory vasoconstriction (oligemia related to cortical spreading depression), intracerebral large-vessel spasm, and vascular endothelium-related hypercoagulability. Results from prospective data indicate that migraine without aura has a lower risk of ischemic vascular events than does migraine with aura.[10]

Cluster headaches have many similarities to migraine attacks, but there are several distinguishing clinical and pathophysiological features. Strict circadian patterns and seasonal occurrence have always suggested hypothalamic involvement, and recent volumetric studies have shown increased gray matter volume in a small region in the posterior hypothalamus. Positron emission tomography and functional magnetic resonance imaging scans showed activation of this area during an attack.[11] Activation of the trigeminovascular system, which leads to secondary hyperfunction of the parasympathetic nervous system, is also unique to cluster headaches.

References

1. Ramadan NM, Halvorson H, Vande-Linde A, et al. Low brain magnesium in migraine. *Headache*. 1989;29:590–593.

2. Trauninger A, Pfund Z, Koszegi T, Czopf J. Oral magnesium load test in patients with migraine. *Headache*. 2002;42:114–119.

3. Mauskop A, Altura BT, Cracco RQ, Altura BM: Deficiency in serum ionized Mg but not total Mg in patients with migraine. Possible role of ICa^{2+}/IMg^{2+} ratio. *Headache*. 1993;33(3):135–138.

4. Weiller C, May A, Limmroth V, et al. Brain stem activation in spontaneous human migraine attacks. *Nat Med*. 1995;1:658–660.

5. Burstein R, Cutrer MF, Yarnitsky D. The development of cutaneous allodynia during a migraine attack: Clinical evidence for the sequential recruitment of spinal and supraspinal nociceptive neurons in migraine. *Brain*. 2000;123:1703–1709.

6. Hadjikhani N, Sanchez Del Rio M, Wu O, et al. Mechanisms of migraine aura revealed by functional MRI in human visual cortex. *Proc Natl Acad Sci U S A*. 2001;98:4687–4892.

7. Goadsby PJ. Recent advances in understanding migraine mechanisms, molecules and therapeutics. *Trends Mol Med*. 2007;13:39–44.

8. Edvinsson L. Novel migraine therapy with calcitonin gene-regulated peptide receptor antagonists. *Exp Opin Therap Targets*. 2007;11:1179–1188.

9. Olesen J, Diener HC, Husstedt IW, et al. Calcitonin gene-related peptide receptor antagonist BIBN 4096 BS for the acute treatment of migraine. *N Engl J Med*. 2004;350:1104–1110.

10. Etminan M, Takkouche B, Isorna FC, Samii A. Risk of ischaemic stroke in people with migraine: Systematic review and meta-analysis of observational studies. *BMJ*. 2005;330:54–55.

11. Dasilva AF, Goadsby PJ, Borsook D: Cluster headache: A review of neuroimaging findings. *Curr Pain Headache Rep*. 2007;11:131–136.

Chapter 3

Diagnostic Procedures

Taking a good history is necessary to making any medical diagnosis, but this is particularly true in neurology and even more so in dealing with patients with headaches. The aspects of history that need to be elicited include circumstances surrounding the onset of headaches, duration, frequency, time patterns, possible aggravating and relieving factors, preceding and associated symptoms, quality and distribution of pain, prior treatments attempted, and coexistent medical conditions. Social history can reveal job-related stress, working conditions, occupational triggers, family problems, living conditions, and other factors that may worsen headaches. Information about alcohol and caffeine consumption, smoking, diet, sleep, and exercise is also highly relevant. Family history often provides invaluable clues, such as history of similar headaches, early strokes and coronary artery disease, mental illness, and so on. A thorough physical examination is the next stop in patient evaluation and can reveal, in addition to neurological abnormalities, neck muscle spasm, tenderness of temporo-mandibular joints, poor posture, and so on. An examination should also look for loss of vibration sense in patients' feet—an early sign of a peripheral neuropathy often due to vitamin B12 deficiency, which can worsen headaches, cause fatigue, and other symptoms. Imaging studies and other tests make the smallest contribution in establishing the diagnosis and are generally overused.

Blood Tests

The presence of symptoms suggesting an underlying medical problem warrants further investigation, including a battery of blood tests. Hypothyroidism can occasionally present with headache as the only symptom or with nonspecific symptoms such as malaise, fatigue, and constipation. It can occur in women after delivery or without any obvious trigger. C-reactive protein (CRP) and erythrocyte sedimentation rate (ESR) help detect the presence of temporal arteritis, with CRP being a more sensitive and reliable test. Anemia, collagen-vascular conditions, Lyme disease, HIV, and other infections can present with headaches, but usually other symptoms are also present. Serum and particularly red blood cell magnesium levels can be helpful. Vitamin B_{12} deficiency does not usually cause headaches, but it can be a contributing factor. It should be considered in patients who are vegetarians and those with irritable bowel syndrome, frequent diarrhea, or other causes of malabsorption. Checking homocysteine levels may help identify patients who should be treated with vitamins B12, B6, and folate. S. Wheeler discovered vitamin D deficiency in 42% of patients with chronic migraines, although it is not clear that supplementation with vitamin D relieves headaches.

Magnetic Resonance Imaging

According to the guidelines of the American Academy of Neurology,[1] brain imaging studies are not required in patients with typical migraine headaches who have no symptoms of another disease and who have a normal physical examination. However, in practice we use magnetic resonance imaging (MRI) scans much more often than necessary for diagnostic reasons. Scans are often done to allay patients' fears, and some patients obtain therapeutic benefit from an MRI scan—they stop worrying about having a brain tumor, and this leads to improvement in their headaches. Table 3.1 provides appropriate reasons to obtain MRI. MRI is a much better test than a computed tomography (CT) scan for evaluation of headaches, because CT scans can miss white matter abnormalities, pituitary adenoma, Chiari malformation, and other posterior fossa abnormalities. Drawbacks of MRI include higher cost, claustrophobic experience, and, unlike with CT, exaggerated appearance of inflammatory changes in paranasal sinuses. The latter often leads to an erroneous diagnosis of sinus headaches, which are already overdiagnosed. CT also has an advantage over MRI in the early diagnosis of an acute intracranial hemorrhage. However, radiation exposure from CT is not trivial and is another reason to favor MRI.

White matter abnormalities are seen on MRI in about 10% of migraine sufferers. These are usually small, are scattered throughout the brain, and are of uncertain significance. A report by T. Rozen documented the disappearance of a white matter lesion within a few days after the initial MRI scan, suggesting that these may be due to functional rather than structural abnormalities.[2] This should not be surprising, because we do not see accumulation of these lesions over the years. However, these lesions do cause anxiety in many patients, particularly if they read the differential diagnosis offered by the radiologist, which includes demyelinating and cerebrovascular disease. Clinical correlation, personal review of the images, and a discussion with the neuroradiologist are sometimes necessary, as multiple sclerosis and other conditions can obviously occur in migraine sufferers.

Table 3.1 When to obtain an MRI
• Recent onset of severe headaches
• Patient is very anxious and has not had a scan recently
• Sudden change in headache frequency, severity, or character
• Worst headache of one's life
• First episode of exertional or sex-induced headache
• Typical primary headache that does not respond to treatment
• Presence of neck stiffness, fever, or any neurological signs and symptoms

Magnetic Resonance Venography and Magnetic Resonance Angiography

Patients with sudden onset of severe headaches (usually with focal symptoms or papilledema) and with no obvious trigger should be evaluated with magnetic resonance venography (MRV) for possible intracranial venous thrombosis. A suspected intracranial aneurysm or arteritis is diagnosed by magnetic resonance angiography (MRA) and traditional angiography. Acute onset of unilateral headache with neck pain may indicate carotid artery dissection, which can be detected by MRA.

Positron Emission Tomography and Magnetoencephalography

Positron emission tomography (PET) and magnetoencephalography (MEG) have become available commercially; however, they have no proven utility in evaluating headache patients.

Lumbar Puncture

This procedure can be used to diagnose meningitis, high or low intracranial pressure, and subarachnoid hemorrhage. Subarachnoid hemorrhage can be missed by a CT scan in 5% of patients within the first 24 hours and in a higher percentage if the CT scan is done later. Long duration of headaches does not preclude the need for a lumbar puncture. Chronic meningitis can be caused by tuberculosis, borreliosis, syphilis, toxoplasmosis, and other infections. Obesity, with or very rarely without papilledema, is an indication for a lumbar puncture, which can establish the diagnosis of pseudotumor cerebri, also termed benign intracranial hypertension. Abrupt onset of headaches with increased intracranial pressure should lead to MRV to look for cerebral venous thrombosis. The diagnosis of low cerebrospinal fluid pressure headaches can usually be established on the basis of a typical clinical presentation and characteristic MRI scan findings (meningeal enhancement on a contrast-enhanced MRI), without the need for a lumbar puncture.

Electroencephalography

This procedure is rarely useful because subclinical or nocturnal seizures as a cause of headaches without other symptoms are rare occurrences. However, if a patient has a history of head injury or a focal, even if static, brain lesion, epilepsy should be considered. Also keep in mind that epilepsy and migraine are comorbid conditions, so having one condition increases the risk of having the other. The preferred test is an ambulatory 24-hour electroencephalography, which is more likely to capture epileptic activity than the standard 20-minute recording.

Neuropsychological Evaluation

Complaints of poor memory are very common among patients with chronic or frequent migraine attacks. This is likely to be due to the disruptive effect of pain on memory processes and the psychological stress patients may be under. Memory usually improves with the relief of headaches. Neuropsychological evaluation is not necessary except in patients with post-traumatic headaches in whom the injury may also cause cognitive impairment.

Electrocardiography, Stress Test, Coronary Angiography, and Sleep Study

An electrocardiogram is indicated in some patients being treated with tricyclic antidepressants, methadone, and calcium channel blockers, since these drugs can cause cardiac conduction problems. This test should be obtained in patients before escalation of the dose or when cardiac risk factors are present. Patients with risk factors for coronary artery disease who are being considered for treatment with triptans should be evaluated for coronary artery disease at least with a nuclear exercise stress test and possibly coronary angiography, depending on the risk factors present.

A sleep study is used to diagnose restless leg syndrome, sleep apnea, and other sleep disorders that impair quality of sleep and can worsen migraine and tension-type headaches. Sleep disorders are particularly common in patients with cluster headaches.[3]

References

1. Practice parameter: Evidence-based guidelines for migraine headache (an evidence-based review): Report of the Quality Standards Subcommittee of the American Academy of Neurology. *Neurology.* 2000;55:754–762.

2. Rozen TD. Vanishing cerebellar infarcts in a migraine patient. *Cephalalgia.* 2007; 27:557–560.

3. Nobre ME, Filho PFM, Dominici M. Cluster headache associated with sleep apnoea. *Cephalalgia.* 2003;23:276–279.

Chapter 4

Nonpharmacological/ Alternative Approaches

It may seem unnecessary to tell patients to get enough sleep, exercise, eat at regular intervals, and drink enough water, but a significant number of patients will in fact listen to the physician and modify their habits. Many migraine patients do much better if they adhere to a strict routine in regard to their sleep, food intake, and exercise.

What about all those "alternative" therapies that many physicians disdain? The National Center for Complementary and Alternative Medicine (CAM) of the National Institutes of Health (NIH) defines CAM as "a group of diverse medical and health care systems, practices, and products that are not presently considered to be part of conventional medicine." A more appropriate term, which encompasses the use of these therapies, is integrative medicine. The use of nontraditional therapies in migraine is increasing, with the amount of money spent on such therapies surpassing that spent for inpatient treatment within the United States. Because more and more patients are turning to such therapies, physicians need to be aware of the types of alternative treatments that their patients may be receiving.

It is estimated that current pharmacological options are not effective for over 30% of headache patients. In addition, research has shown poor compliance with prophylactic migraine regimens, undermining their potential efficacy. A covert observational study found a compliance rate of only 66% with a once-daily dosing regimen, and lower rates with regimens requiring multiple doses each day.

Cognitive Techniques

Many people feel that they do not have time to engage in cognitive techniques. They seem to miss the irony—the busier they are, the more they would benefit from meditation and relaxation training. Cognitive and behavioral techniques can produce a change from external to internal locus of control. This makes people feel less helpless in the face of their illness and stress, and allows them to gain some measure of control over their condition. The most widely used behavioral treatments for headache include progressive relaxation, biofeedback, cognitive-behavioral techniques, and stress-management therapies. These approaches can be used in combination with pharmacological and other non-drug therapies. The purpose of relaxation and biofeedback training is to enable patients to recognize and learn to control headache-related physiological responses. As Ken Holroyd puts it, the goals of cognitive-behavioral therapy are to enable patients to identify and manage thoughts and beliefs that can trigger or maintain headaches.[1] Cognitive techniques can also help improve adherence to therapeutic regimens. Table 4.1 provides a list of goals of cognitive-behavioral therapy. Reasons for nonadherence are listed in Table 4.2, as outlined by Steven Baskin.

While self-taught relaxation techniques can be equally effective, biofeedback offers the advantage of having a personal coach teaching, motivating, and supervising the process. As few as three biofeedback sessions can be effective, although a typical course involves about 10 sessions. The sessions consist of learning relaxation and breathing techniques, which allow the patient to learn to control physiological functions that are normally not under conscious control. Feedback from a temperature or electromyography probe is typically displayed on a computer monitor. Patients are often impressed by their new-found ability to control the action on a computer screen purely by thought. With regular practice patients may not need to rely on visual feedback, and become able to control tension in their body without effort. Biofeedback has been shown to be effective for both migraine and tension-type headaches. In one biofeedback study with five-year follow-up, 80% to 90% of migraine and tension-type headache patients reported continued benefit following a single course of biofeedback.[2]

Table 4.1 Goals of cognitive-behavioral therapy

- Attempt to foster an internal locus of control and modify distress-related thoughts
- Rehearse adaptive cognitive and behavioral responses to the development of a migraine
- Accurately interpret body signals
- Develop action plans
- Reduce anxiety and depression
- Recognize triggers

Table 4.2 Nonadherence to therapeutic regimens

- Lack of money
- Lack of insight
- Poor instructions
- Unrealistic expectations
- Strong belief systems ("I don't need medicine")
- Psychiatric comorbidity
- Helplessness, pessimism, affective distress
- Anger at health care provider
- Complex therapies require changes in behavior

Physical Methods

Cardiovascular or aerobic exercise is arguably one of the best prophylactic treatments for migraine and tension-type headaches. Often it is necessary to explain to a skeptical patient how exercise might help. With varying degrees of scientific accuracy, these are three sufficiently convincing reasons why exercise can help: It is relaxing before or after a stressful day, it improves circulation in the brain, and it releases endorphins—intrinsic pain-relieving substances. Until recently, this recommendation came from anecdotal observations, but a group of Swedish researchers examined records of over 46,000 people that showed an inverse correlation between exercise and headaches of any type.[3] The same group conducted a controlled study in 91 migraine patients comparing aerobic exercise 40 minutes three times a week with topiramate and with progressive relaxation. All three treatment groups did equally well.[4]

Physical therapy can be very effective for cervicogenic headaches, which are more common in the elderly and after injuries. If physical therapy is not practical for financial or logistical reasons, a simple set of neck exercises combined with regular aerobic exercise or yoga can be very effective. The most effective neck exercise is isometric strengthening of the neck muscles, which should be done very frequently throughout the day to produce the desired effect (see Figure 4.1).

While massage is a pleasant and often helpful treatment, it is also expensive and impractical, because many sessions are needed to achieve meaningful results. Some patients report that reaching an orgasm relieves their migraine attack, although many would probably have difficulty doing that while having a headache. Release of endorphins is the likely mechanism.

Chiropractic intervention, particularly high-velocity adjustment, carries a small but not negligible risk of carotid or vertebral artery dissection or subdural hematoma. A variety of other forms of manual therapy (craniosacral, Feldenkrais, Alexander) can be effective in some patients. Improper posture can cause neck and shoulder strain, which in turn can worsen migraine or cause tension-type headache.

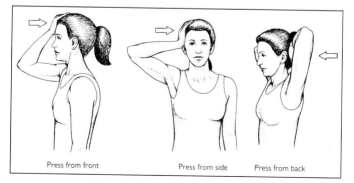

Press from front   Press from side   Press from back

Figure 4.1 Isometric exercise

Dental appliances can help patients with malocclusion, clenching, or bruxism. In addition to headaches, these patients often experience pain in the jaw. These appliances are more likely to help if the patient has pain or tenderness of the temporomandibular joints. A typical full bite plate may prevent tooth wear but will not prevent clenching, and probably is not as effective as a partial device, which covers only the front teeth (Nociceptive Trigeminal Inhibition device [NTI], Best-Bite). A review of five randomized controlled trials showed that the NTI device was beneficial for temporomandibular disorders and headaches[5]. The NTI device is custom-made by a dentist and is worn during sleep and stressful times during the day. Prolonged use of the NTI device can cause malocclusion, which can be severe and at times can develop after only a few months of wear. The NTI device also carries the risk of being swallowed or chocked upon. Another device, Best-Bite, is worn only during the day and is not likely to cause malocclusion; however, it is visible and can only be worn in private.

Acupuncture

A 1997 National Institutes of Health consensus statement supported acupuncture as a legitimate therapy with proven efficacy for adult postoperative dental pain and chemotherapy-induced nausea. It also suggested possible efficacy as either adjunctive therapy or as an acceptable alternative deserving additional investigation for a variety of other painful conditions including headache. A systematic review of randomized controlled trials of true and sham acupuncture for migraines and tension-type headaches found that eight trials showed statistical superiority of true treatment, four showed a trend toward superiority, and two showed no difference.[6] These findings were supported by a recent randomized trial in 401 patients with chronic headaches.[7] The German government sponsored what can be considered a definitive study of acupuncture in headaches, which involved 15,056 headache patients.[8] The authors of this study concluded that "acupuncture plus routine care in patients with headache was associated with marked clinical improvements compared with routine care alone." Limiting factors for wider use of acupuncture are its cost and time commitment. A typical course of acupuncture involves 10 or more weekly sessions and involves placement of 10 to 30 needles. The exact placement of needles, based on theories of traditional Chinese medicine, does not appear to be critical for the success of treatment. A simplified approach, which can be easily learned by any interested health care provider, yields similar benefits. Potential complications of acupuncture, most of which can be avoided, include transmission of infection by nonsterile needles, pneumothorax, syncope, and hematoma.

Magnesium

Magnesium plays an integral role in the pathogenesis of migraines. Glutamate, calcitonin gene-related peptide (CGRP), acetylcholine, nitric oxide, norepinephrine, potassium, calcium, 325 enzyme complexes, angiotensin II, serotonin, and G proteins are all influenced by magnesium concentration.

A 1989 NMR spectroscopy study by N. Ramadan showed decreased magnesium levels in brains of patients with migraines compared with control subjects.[9] Migraine patients were also found to have low serum and tissue levels of magnesium in many other studies. A study conducted by a group of Hungarian researchers led by T. Trauninger showed that migraine patients had a systemic magnesium deficiency by giving an oral loading dose of magnesium and measuring 24-hour urinary magnesium excretion.[10] Potential causes of magnesium deficiency include stress, genetic factors, low dietary intake, gastrointestinal disorders, alcohol, and chronic illness. A significant drop in ionized and total plasma levels of magnesium was observed under conditions of chronic emotional stress.[11] It is possible that magnesium depletion is the biological mechanism of stress-induced headaches. Hangover headaches could be also due to depletion of magnesium by alcohol.

A study of 40 consecutive migraine patients by this author and his colleagues found that intravenous treatment with magnesium sulfate provides very good and sustained relief to more than 50% of patients within 15 minutes of infusion.[12] Further analysis showed that 86% of patients who responded to magnesium had low pretreatment serum ionized magnesium levels, in contrast to only 16% of nonresponders. Very similar results were obtained in patients with cluster headaches.[13] Of 22 cluster headache patients, 40% responded with the resolution of their cluster period. The responders had low ionized magnesium levels, while nonresponders had normal levels.

Two double-blind studies found positive results with oral magnesium supplementation.[14,15] The first study, performed in Italian women by F. Facchinetti and his colleagues, showed that in addition to the reduction in number of migraine days (4.7 versus 2.4, p < 0.01), symptoms of premenstrual distress were also relieved. The second study of 81 German migraine patients conducted by a group led by A. Peikert showed that attack frequency was reduced in 41.6% of patients taking 600 mg of trimagnesium dicitrate daily, compared to 15.8% (p < 0.05) of patients taking placebo. Days with migraine were reduced in 52.3% of patients on magnesium and 19.5% of patients on placebo (p < 0.05). Negative findings of a third study have been attributed to the choice of a magnesium formulation that was poorly absorbed and resulted in diarrhea in 45% of patients.[16] A double-blind study of magnesium supplementation in children by F. Wang and colleagues did not unequivocally determine whether oral magnesium oxide is superior to placebo in preventing frequent migrainous headache in children, but treatment with the active agent did lead to a significant reduction in headache days.[17] Another interesting study by R. Cady found that patients who did not respond to sumatriptan had low ionized magnesium levels. They became responders after taking a magnesium supplement.

Serum magnesium levels do not provide an accurate reflection of the amount of magnesium in the body, because only 1–2% of magnesium in the body is extracellular. Drs. Burton and Bella Altura of the State University of

New York, Downstate Medical Center, are responsible for a major advance in magnesium research, in part by developing an ion-selective electrode to measure ionized magnesium levels.[18] These levels are much more accurate than serum levels and have been used for many pioneering studies in headaches and other fields. The test for ionized magnesium levels is not available commercially, although the test for red blood cell (RBC) levels of magnesium is available and offers a better measure than the serum levels. Considering that (1) the cost of measuring RBC magnesium level is about $80, (2) a one-month supply of magnesium oxide at a dose of 400 mg a day costs less than two dollars, and (3) half of migraine sufferers could benefit, it is reasonable to start magnesium supplementation in all patients with migraine without testing. Because oral magnesium supplements sometimes are not well absorbed, an intravenous infusion can be both therapeutic and diagnostic. If a positive response occurs, oral supplementation is started. The response to the infusion given during an attack to a patient deficient in magnesium is dramatic. The infusion can be done using one g of magnesium sulfate in 10 mL of normal saline by slow push over five minutes using a butterfly needle. Relief begins before the end of infusion, and within minutes, the patient feels significant improvement. The author has performed this infusion in thousands of patients and the only side effects encountered in a small number of patients have been nausea and dizziness.

Other symptoms that can suggest the presence of magnesium deficiency include coldness of extremities (or just generally always feeling cold), leg muscle cramps, and premenstrual syndrome. Patients should be started on 400 mg of magnesium oxide daily. If necessary, and if tolerated, this dose can be increased to 800 mg, and even 1,200 mg in divided doses. The only potential side effect of oral magnesium is stomach pain and diarrhea, especially if it is taken on an empty stomach. Should this occur, a different form of magnesium (chelated, slow-release, liquid) can be administered. A small percentage of patients need monthly infusions of magnesium. This group includes patients who do not tolerate oral magnesium, do not absorb it, or do not remember to take it. If magnesium is taken with calcium, calcium can reduce the absorption of magnesium, while magnesium enhances the absorption of calcium. Magnesium is excreted by kidneys and therefore should be used with caution (i.e., with frequent blood tests) in patients with renal failure.

α-Lipoic Acid

α-Lipoic or thioctic acid has been studied for the prevention of migraine headaches in a single trial in Belgium.[19] Intent-to-treat analysis was performed in 44 patients enrolled in the study. Monthly attack frequency tended to be reduced between run-in and the third month of treatment in the thioctic acid group compared to placebo ($p = 0.06$). The proportion of 50% responders was not significantly different between thioctic acid (30.8%) and placebo (27.8%).

Within-group analyses showed a significant reduction of attack frequency ($p = 0.005$), headache days ($p = 0.009$), and headache severity ($p = 0.03$) in patients treated with thioctic acid for three months, while these outcome measures remained unchanged in the placebo group. No adverse effects were reported. The dose used in this study was 600 mg daily.

Coenzyme Q_{10}

Coenzyme Q_{10} (CoQ_{10}) is an essential element of the mitochondrial electron transport chain and is vital in energy metabolism. CoQ_{10}, 100 mg, three times a day was compared with placebo in 42 migraine patients in a double-blind, randomized, placebo-controlled trial conducted by P. Sandor and his colleagues in Switzerland.[20] CoQ_{10} was superior to placebo for attack frequency, headache days, and days with nausea in the third treatment month; the 50% responder rate for attack frequency was 14.4% for placebo and 47.6% for CoQ_{10}. The treatment was well tolerated.

A.D. Hershey and his collaborators conducted a study to assess the role of CoQ_{10} deficiency and supplementation in a large group of children with migraines.[21] CoQ_{10} was measured in 1,550 children, mostly adolescents. Of these patients, 32.9% were below the reference range. Children with low CoQ_{10} were started on one to three mg/kg per day of CoQ_{10} in liquid gel capsule formulation. In a subset of patients who returned for timely follow-up (mean, 97 days), the total CoQ_{10} level improved ($p < 0.0001$), while the headache frequency improved from 19.2 to 12.5 ($p < 0.001$) and headache disability assessed with PedMIDAS improved from 47.4 to 22.8 ($p < 0.001$). The optimal dose of CoQ_{10} remains to be determined, and judging by a study performed in patients with Parkinson's disease, it may be significantly higher than 300 mg a day. In this dose-ranging, double-blind, placebo-controlled, nine-month-long study, only the highest dosage of 1200 mg a day provided significant relief of symptoms of Parkinson's disease compared to placebo. [22]

Riboflavin

Riboflavin, or vitamin B_2, which has a function similar to CoQ_{10} in that it also improves energy metabolism, has also been studied for the prevention of migraine by J. Schoenen and colleagues in Belgium.[23] The study involved 55 patients who received a daily intake of either 400 mg of riboflavin or placebo for three months. Fifty-nine percent of the patients receiving riboflavin improved by at least 50%, versus 15% patients on placebo ($p = 0.002$). Riboflavin was also found to be superior to placebo in reducing attack frequency ($p = 0.005$) and number of headache days ($p = 0.012$). The difference with placebo appeared only on the third month.

Herbal Remedies

A variety of herbal remedies have been reported to prevent headaches in some patients. The major difficulty in studying herbal remedies is the natural variation in the amount of active ingredients, most of which are yet to be defined. Plants grown in different conditions and processed differently will yield differing amounts of active ingredients. The nature and the number of these ingredients are not clear, making standardization difficult. Nevertheless, feverfew and butterbur are two common plants that have been in use for many years and recently have been proven to be effective in preventing migraine headaches. Unfortunately, herbal products are not regulated in the United States. However, they are in Germany, and German physicians have been in the vanguard of research on herbal products. Advise your patients to buy products manufactured by major manufacturers, where quality control is likely to be high. Some of these manufacturers include Puritan's Pride, GNC, Centrum, Nature Made, Solgar, Carlson, and CVS.

Feverfew

Feverfew (*Tanacetum parthenium*) has been studied in several randomized, double-blind, placebo-controlled trials, in which it was shown to afford prophylaxis against migraine versus placebo. In one study, patients receiving feverfew experienced a statistically significant reduction in the mean number and severity of attacks, and in the degree of nausea and vomiting; however, feverfew had no significant effect on the duration of attacks.[24] The most definitive study, performed by H.C. Diener and his colleagues in Germany in 170 patients, used feverfew subjected to a highly sophisticated extraction method, and this study showed reduction in number of attacks in a 28-day period, improvement in global assessment of efficacy, and no difference in adverse events compared to placebo.[25] The treatment had no effect on duration of attacks. It appears that feverfew is an effective prophylactic agent in the treatment of migraines. Side effects attributed to feverfew include mouth sores and allergic reactions.

Butterbur

Butterbur (*Petasites hybridus*) is a common plant that contains dangerous toxins. A single manufacturer has succeeded in purifying the extract of the root of this plant, with the commercial product proved to be safe in standard animal essays for teratogenicity and carcinogenicity. A double-blind, placebo-controlled, randomized trial performed by R. Lipton, this author, and their colleagues with 245 patients showed migraine attack frequency reduction of 48% in the 150 mg group (p = 0.0012) and 36% in the 100 mg group (p = 0.127) against 26% in the placebo group.[26] The product was very well tolerated, with the only common side effect being burping with an unpleasant smell. It is available in 50 and 75 mg tablets.

Table 4.3 Supplements for the prevention of migraines

Supplement	Daily dose	Side effects	Comments
Magnesium	400 mg	Diarrhea, stomach pain	Various magnesium salts may have fewer gastrointestinal side effects and better absorption
Coenzyme Q$_{10}$	300 mg	Stomach upset, insomnia	Doses of 1200 mg are used for Parkinson's disease with few side effects
Riboflavin	400 mg	Bright yellow urine color	Urine color is not really a side effect, but can alarm some patients
Feverfew	100 mg	Mouth sores, upset stomach, allergic reaction	Amount of active ingredients varies among products
Butterbur	150 mg	Burping up unpleasant taste, allergic reaction	Caution patients against homemade butterbur products—the plant is toxic and only one manufacturer (Weber & Weber) makes a safe product
α-Lipoic (thioctic) acid	600 mg	Stomach pain, allergic reaction	

References

1. Holroyd KA, Mauskop A: Complementary and alternative treatments. *Neurology.* 2003;60(suppl 2):S58–S62.

2. Blanchard EB, Appelbaum KA, Guarnieri P, Morrill B, Dentinger MP. Five year prospective follow-up on the treatment of chronic headache with biofeedback and/or relaxation. *Headache.* 1987;27:580–583.

3. Varkey E, Hagen K, Zwart J-A, Linde M. Physical activity and headache: results from the Nord-Trøndelag Health Study (HUNT). *Cephalalgia* 2008;28:1292–1297.

4. Varkey E, Cider A, J. Carlsson J, Linde M. Exercise as migraine prophylaxis: A randomized study using relaxation and topiramate as controls. *Cephalalgia* 2011;31:1428–1438.

5. Stapelmann H, Turp JC. The NTI-tss device for the therapy of bruxism, temporo-mandibular disorders, and headache: Where do we stand? A qualitative systematic review of the literature. *BMC Oral Health.* 2008;8:22.

6. Melchart D, Linde K, Fischer P, et al. Acupuncture for recurrent headaches: A systematic review of randomized controlled trials. *Cephalalgia.* 1999;19:779–786.

7. Vickers AJ, Rees, RW, Zollman, CE, et al. Acupuncture for chronic headache in primary care: Large, pragmatic, randomised trial. *BMJ.* 2004;328:744.

8. Jena S, Witt CM, Brinkhaus B, Wegscheider K, Willich SN. Acupuncture in patients with headache. *Cephalalgia.* 2008;28:969–979.

9. Ramadan NM, Halvorson H, Vande-Linde A, et al. Low brain magnesium in migraine. *Headache.* 1989;29:590–593.

10. Trauninger A, Pfund Z, Koszegi T, Czopf J. Oral magnesium load test in patients with migraine. *Headache*. 2002;42:114–119.

11. Cernak I, Savic V, Kotur J, Prokic V, Kuljic B, Grbovic D, Veljovic M. Alterations in magnesium and oxidative status during chronic emotional stress. *Magnes Res.* 2000;13(1):29–36.

12. Mauskop A, Altura BT, Cracco RQ, Altura BM. Intravenous magnesium sulfate relieves migraine attacks in patients with low serum ionized magnesium levels: A pilot study. *Clin Sci.* 1995;89:633–636.

13. Mauskop A, Altura BT, Cracco RQ, Altura BM: Intravenous magnesium sulfate relieves cluster headaches in patients with low serum ionized magnesium levels. *Headache* 1995;35:597–600.

14. Facchinetti F, Sances G, Genazzani AR, Nappi G. Magnesium prophylaxis of menstrual migraine: Effects on intracellular magnesium. *Headache*. 1991;31:298–301.

15. Peikert A, Wilimzig C, Kohne-Volland R. Prophylaxis of migraine with oral magnesium: Results from a prospective, multicenter, placebo-controlled and double-blind randomized study. *Cephalalgia*. 1996;16:257–263.

16. Pfaffenrath V, Wessely P, Meyer C, et al. Magnesium in the prophylaxis of migraine: A double-blind, placebo-controlled study. *Cephalalgia*. 1996;16:436–440.

17. Wang F, Van Den Eeden SK, Ackerson LM, Salk SE, Reince RH, Elin RJ. Oral magnesium oxide prophylaxis of frequent migrainous headache in children: A randomized, double-blind, placebo-controlled trial. *Headache*. 2003;43:601–610.

18. Altura BT, Shirley T, Young CC, Dell'Ofrano K, Handwerker SM, Altura BM. A new method for the rapid determination of ionized Mg2+ in whole blood, serum and plasma. *Meth Find Exp Clin Pharmacol*. 1992;14:297–304.

19. Magis D, Ambrosini A, Sándor P, Jacquy J, Laloux P Schoenen J. A randomized double-blind placebo-controlled trial of thioctic acid in migraine prophylaxis. *Headache*. 2007;47:52–57.

20. Sándor PS, DiClemente L, Coppola G. Efficacy of coenzyme Q10 in migraine prophylaxis: A randomized controlled trial. *Neurology*. 2005;64:713–715.

21. Hershey AD, Powers SW, Vockell ALB, et al. Coenzyme Q10 deficiency and response to supplementation in pediatric and adolescent migraine. *Headache*. 2007;47:73–80.

22. Shults CW, Oakes D, Kieburtz K, et al. Effects of coenzyme Q10 in early parkinson disease evidence of slowing of the functional decline. *Arch Neurol*. 2002;59(10):1541–1550.

23. Schoenen J, Jacquy J, Lenaerts M. High dose riboflavin is effective in migraine prophylaxis: Results of a double-blind, randomized placebo-controlled trial. *Neurology*. 1998;50:446–470.

24. Murphy JJ, Heptinsall S, Mitchell JRA. Randomized double-blind placebo-controlled trial of feverfew in migraine prevention. *Lancet*. 1988;23:189–192.

25. Diener HC, Pfaffenrath V, Schnitker J, et al. Efficacy and safety of 6.25 mg t.i.d. feverfew CO2-extract (MIG-99) in migraine prevention—A randomized, double-blind, multicentre, placebo-controlled study. *Cephalalgia*. 2005;25:1031–1041.

26. Lipton RB, Gobel H, Einhaupl KM, Wilks K, Mauskop A. *Petasites hybridus* root (butterbur) is an effective preventive treatment for migraine. *Neurology*. 2004;63:2240–2244.

Chapter 5

Pharmacological Therapies

General Guidelines for the Use of Abortive Agents

Abortive medications are used to stop an individual attack, while prophylactic drugs are taken daily to prevent attacks from occurring. Some drugs, such as nonsteroidal anti-inflammatory agents (NSAIDs), can be used for both abortive and prophylactic therapy. Mini-prophylaxis refers to the daily use of abortive drugs, such as triptans or NSAIDs, (as well as prophylactic drugs) for several days or a week to prevent an expected (usually menstrual) attack.

When deciding on acute treatment, results of past treatments, frequency of attacks, severity and types of attacks, and presence of other medical conditions should be considered. Relief of pain and associated symptoms with return to normal functioning is the goal. An additional goal is overall improvement in the quality of life. With this goal in mind, the vast majority of migraine patients seeing a physician should receive a triptan as the first choice of therapy, unless triptans are contraindicated. This is the case because by the time patients decide to seek care for their headaches, most have tried over-the-counter analgesics and have at least a moderate level of disability.

The stratified approach to abortive care means treating milder headaches with an NSAID, while using a triptan for more severe attacks. Another approach to stratified care is to use the MIDAS score (see chapter 7). If the disability score is six or higher, use a triptan. The stepwise approach advocates using an NSAID before proceeding to a triptan in every case. It is surprising how many patients adhere to the stepwise approach even when an NSAID never works. They keep expecting relief, but invariably have to take a stronger drug, which would be more effective if taken early. Many patients recognize that they have a narrow window when the abortive medication can completely abort their migraine attack. However, some patients are not aware that such a window exists. These patients often wait to take their medication, especially if it is a prescription drug and especially if the number of pills they get from their insurance is limited or they have to pay for it. Frequently, these patients will not only obtain much better control of their headaches, but will also need fewer tablets per attack if the medication is taken early. This strategy is a little more problematic in patients with frequent attacks. Some patients are so anxious about not missing this window of opportunity that they will take the medication even when they are not certain if a headache is coming. This can lead to medication overuse headaches, a phenomenon shown to occur commonly with caffeine, butalbital, or an opioid, but very rarely with triptans or NSAIDs. The accepted limit for medications with caffeine, butalbital, or opioids is that they should be taken on not more than two days a week, even if more than one tablet is taken on those days. This is not a hard and fast rule, and some patients do well taking abortive drugs more frequently, especially when treating menstrual attacks, which can last for up to a week and require daily medication.

Patients often need to treat two or three attacks to judge the efficacy of a particular drug, unless, of course, it caused side effects or worsening of symptoms on the first try. On the follow-up visits it is important to inquire about the efficacy, side effects, and overall impression of the medication. The patient may be ecstatic about finally getting some pain relief, but in fact the functioning may be still impaired due to persistent nausea or drug side effects, and the treatment can be further improved by trying a different triptan or different route of its administration, by adding an antiemetic or an NSAID, or by treating headaches earlier.

Nonsteroidal Anti-Inflammatory Drugs

NSAIDs, such as ibuprofen (Advil, Advil-Migraine, Motrin), diclofenac (Voltaren), naproxen (Naprosyn, Anaprox), aspirin, aspirin/magnesium combination (Migralex), and, to a lesser extent, acetaminophen (Tylenol), are effective for tension-type and milder migraine headaches.[1] While parenteral ketorolac is an effective analgesic, oral ketorolac provides pain relief not any greater than provided by ibuprofen or aspirin. However, its gastrointestinal side effects are much more severe, and this drug should not be used in oral form. Two tablets containing a combination of 1,000 mg of aspirin and 150 mg of magnesium oxide (Migralex) possibly offers better efficacy and reduced risk of gastric irritation with rapid onset due to a quick dissolution formula. Magnesium provides additional relief of migraine and also acts as a buffering agent (pH of magnesium oxide is 10), protecting against the gastrointestinal side effects of aspirin. A recent Cochrane review of 13 studies (involving 4,222 patients) which compared the efficacy of 1,000 mg of aspirin and 100 mg of sumatriptan in the treatment of migraines determined that these two drugs had equal efficacy and aspirin (even without magnesium) had fewer side effects.[2] Another popular combination available without prescription is that of aspirin, acetaminophen, and caffeine (Excedrin, Excedrin Migraine). However, caffeine, particularly when added to the dietary intake, has the potential to cause rebound headaches, while caffeine can increase gastrointestinal side effects of aspirin.

Triptans

Patrick Humphrey led the development of a truly revolutionary drug, sumatriptan (Imitrex, Imitrex Nasal Spray, Imitrex Injection, Treximet—sumatriptan with naproxen sodium), which was to become the first in the family of triptans (see Table 5.1). These are so-called designer drugs specifically developed to

Table 5.1 Triptans

Name (Brand/ generic)	Formulations (mg)	Half-life (hours)	2-hour response rate (%)
Almotriptan/Axert	6.25, 12.5*	3	61
Eletriptan/Relpax	20, 40*	5	60 (40 mg)
Frovatriptan/Frova	2.5	26	44
Naratriptan/Amerge	1.25, 2.5*	6	48
Rizatriptan/Maxalt, Maxalt MLT	5, 10* Tablets 5, 10* Orally disintegrating	5	69 (10 mg)
Sumatriptan/Imitrex, Imitrex NS Imitrex Injection Treximet (with naproxen)	25, 50, 100* Tablets 5, 20* Nasal spray 4, 6* Injection 85/500*	2 2/19	62 (100 mg) 61 (20 mg NS) 80 to 85 (6 mg SC) 65
Zolmitriptan/Zomig, Zomig ZMT, Zomig NS	2.5, 5* Tablets 2.5, 5* Orally disintegrating 5* Nasal spray	3	63 (2.5 mg) 70 (5 mg NS)
* Recommended starting dose			

bind to serotonin (5-HT$_{1B}$ and 5-HT$_{1D}$) receptors, which are operational in the development of migraine headaches. Sumatriptan and other triptans are contraindicated in patients with uncontrolled hypertension; history, symptoms, or signs of ischemic cardiac, cerebrovascular, and peripheral vascular syndromes; or basilar and hemiplegic migraines. The diagnosis of basilar migraine is no longer valid, as was mentioned—it is just another term for a migraine with aura. Therefore, the diagnosis of migraine with aura should be made and the triptans can be given. Sumatriptan, rizatriptan, and zolmitriptan should not be given to patients taking monoamine oxidase (MAO) inhibitors. None of the triptans are approved for use in pregnant women and they all belong in Category C, which means that potential side effects should be weighed against potential benefits. Triptan pregnancy registries have collected information on well over 1,000 women who took triptans while pregnant and, so far, no problems have been detected.

Directions for all oral triptans allow taking a second dose two hours after the first one. Injections of sumatriptan can be given one hour apart. Different triptans are not supposed to be taken within 24 hours of each other, although there is no theoretical or experiential reason to prohibit taking a different triptan two hours after another one is taken. The five most effective triptans (all except naratriptan and frovatriptan) have a half-life of two to four hours, so even if one would like to avoid having two triptans on board at the same time, a six-hour interval should suffice. Some physicians even advise their patients to take a short-acting and a long-acting triptan simultaneously—the short-acting provides fast onset of action while the long-acting one prevents the recurrence of pain. This strategy is useful for patients whose headaches keep recurring after taking a short-acting triptan.

Another short-acting triptan, rizatriptan (Maxalt, Maxalt MLT), was developed by Richard Hargreaves and his colleagues. In a meta-analysis of 53 studies involving over 24,000 patients, rizatriptan was shown to be slightly more effective than other triptans.[3] However, the difference among triptans that counts in practice is that each triptan may offer different efficacy and side effects for each individual patient. While the author often begins treatment with sumatriptan (Imitrex) since it is available in a generic form, many patients prefer rizatriptan (Maxalt, Maxalt MLT), zolmitriptan (Zomig, Zomig ZMT, Zomig NS), almotriptan (Axert), or eletriptan (Relpax). Naratriptan (Amerge) has a half-life of six to eight hours and frovatriptan (Frova), 26 hours. These two triptans tend to have slower onset of action and lower overall efficacy, but in practice we find occasional exceptions. Some patients report that after trying all triptans, the fastest-acting and best overall triptan is naratriptan or frovatriptan. The point is that if one triptan is ineffective or causes unpleasant side effects, patients need to try one after another until they can find the best triptan. For many patients, they are all equally effective. The five short-acting ones are much more similar than they are different. All triptans tend to remain effective for long periods of time even if they are taken on a relatively frequent and even daily basis, although the author has encountered patients who stop responding to one triptan after years of use and have to switch to another one.

Combining triptans with NSAID pain relievers may provide better clinical benefit than with either agent alone. A formulation that consists of 85 mg of sumatriptan and 500 mg of naproxen sodium in one tablet (Treximet) offers the convenience of such two drugs in one tablet. In several large studies, administration of this formulation has resulted in two-hour pain-free response in approximately 60% of patients.[4] The combination was more effective than either 100 mg of sumatriptan or 500 mg of naproxen sodium alone.

Daily or frequent use of triptans should be reserved for those rare patients who have failed a multitude of pharmacological and nondrug therapies and for whom triptans allow normal functioning. The question of whether frequent or daily intake of triptans causes rebound (medication overuse) headaches has not been settled. Richard Lipton's year-long observational study suggests that triptans and NSAIDs do not appear to cause worsening of headaches.[5] However, a prophylactic regimen is usually preferred, and physicians should always try to stop daily abortive medications, including triptans. In case of caffeine-containing drugs, this can lead to a quick and dramatic improvement. Withdrawal from barbiturates and opioid drugs has a slower effect. Improvement also happens after withdrawing triptans as well, but the improvement is often less dramatic. The author often gets asked a reasonable question from those few patients who do take triptans daily: Why is it preferable to take a daily prophylactic medication with many more potential side effects? One of the biggest reasons is the cost of triptans, rather than safety. Triptan overuse, unlike that of ergots, was shown not to increase the risk of ischemic complications.[6] Triptans have been in use for over 17 years and have proved to be remarkably safe medications; they are sold without a physician's prescription in Europe.

Another safety issue is that of maximal daily dose of triptans. The current restriction of two doses of the highest strength of all triptans (except for rizatriptan and frovatriptan, where three are allowed) is not based on reliable data. It was derived from the average dose used in clinical trials, rather than daily dose-ranging studies. Considering that most triptans have a short half-life and that in some patients they may have lower bioavailability, it is reasonable to allow a patient an additional dose, especially four to six hours after the last dose.

Potential side effects of triptans include fatigue, dizziness, asthenia, nausea, paresthesias, and neck or chest pressure. The chest pressure sensation is not cardiac in origin and it usually resolves within 15 minutes. If the pressure sensation is mild, with reassurance patients are usually willing to continue taking that particular triptan, but if it is severe or disconcerting, another triptan can be tried.

Administration of Triptans

Sumatriptan injection is available in vials of 4 and 6 mg cartridges for use with an autoinjector (Imitrex), and 6 mg injection pens (Sumavel, Alsuma). Injections can relieve pain, nausea, and other migraine symptoms and allow patients to return to normal functioning within 10 to 20 minutes. Sumatriptan injection can be easily self-administered and its acceptance is surprisingly high, but unfortunately most physicians do not offer it as an option. Sumatriptan injections are also approved for the acute treatment of cluster headaches and have been a true lifesaver to many of those desperate patients. Using sumatriptan in vials allows patients to use a syringe and to inject 2 to 3 mg at a time, which can be effective for some patients with fewer side effects. This is especially useful for cluster patients who can have multiple attacks in one day. Sumatriptan is also available in 25, 50, and 100 mg tablets, in 5 and 20 mg nasal spray, and in tablets containing 85 mg of sumatriptan and 500 mg of naproxen sodium. Side effects are more common with injections and include a flushed sensation, sensation of tightness in the chest, paresthesias, and injection site pain. Nasal spray is the least effective formulation even at 20 mg, while the 5 mg spray is rarely useful. The starting dose of oral sumatriptan for most patients should be 100 mg.

Rizatriptan is available in 5 and 10 mg strengths in a tablet (Maxalt) and as an orally disintegrating tablet (Maxalt MLT). The orally disintegrating formulation is not absorbed in the mouth but needs to descend into the small intestine to get absorbed. It is useful for patients who have difficulty swallowing water because of nausea, when water is not available, or when the patient does not want to appear to be taking a medication. The starting dose of rizatriptan is 10 mg, but when a patient is on propranolol (Inderal), the starting dose is lowered to 5 mg. Some patients believe that the orally disintegrating tablet consistently relieves their headaches much faster than the regular one, sometimes within five minutes. The likely explanation is that the initial relief is due to placebo effect, which is continuously reinforced by the subsequent absorption of the drug and the onset of its real effect, thus producing a Pavlovian conditioning response. There is no point in trying to convince patients that such a prompt response is not possible based on the drug's pharmacokinetics.

Zolmitriptan nasal spray (Zomig NS, 5 mg), anecdotally, is more effective than sumatriptan nasal spray and is a good option for a patient who needs parenteral medication because of severe nausea or who needs rapid onset of action, but who also does not want to resort to sumatriptan injection. Zolmitriptan nasal spray has also been shown to relieve cluster headaches. Zolmitriptan is available in a tablet (Zomig) and orally disintegrating tablet (Zomig ZMT) forms in 2.5 and 5 mg strength.

The orally disintegrating forms of rizatriptan and zolmitriptan contain a small amount of aspartame, which very rarely can cause a headache. Those patients report that their migraine is relieved, but they get a diffuse headache that they might have experienced in the past from aspartame-containing food or drinks. Phenylketonuric patients should not be prescribed these two products.

Naratriptan (Amerge) is a somewhat less effective but a longer-acting triptan. Its half-life is five to eight hours. Naratriptan may be suitable for patients who do not respond to other triptans or for patients whose headaches tend to return within four hours after taking other triptans and for whom multiple doses are required.

Almotriptan (Axert) is available in 6.25 and 12.5 mg tablets and tends to have the lowest incidence of chest pressure sensation.

Eletriptan (Relpax) is available in 20 and 40 mg and, in some European countries, in 80 mg tablets, which supports the notion that the maximal daily limits for triptans are not set in stone and in some patients can be safely exceeded. Eletriptan should not be used within 72 hours of treatment with CYP3A4 inhibitors such as ketoconazole (Nizoral), itraconazole (Sporanox), nefazodone (Serzone), ritonavir (Norvir), nelfinavir (Viracept), clarithromycin (Biaxin), and troleandomycin (TAO).

Frovatriptan (Frova) has a half-life of 26 hours—the longest of all triptans. The tradeoff is slower onset of action, which makes it suitable for patients who have prolonged attacks with slow escalation of pain and other symptoms. Because of its long half-life, frovatriptan is often used for the prevention of menstrual migraines.[7] However, another study showed that sumatriptan 25 mg three times daily and naratriptan 1 mg twice daily are also effective for the prevention of menstrual attacks. These drugs are started one day before the expected headache and are continued throughout the vulnerable period. This finding was replicated in a larger study of naratriptan. Obviously, this strategy works only for women with regular menstrual migraines.

Antiemetics

Antiemetics in the phenothiazine family can relieve not only nausea but, to a certain extent, pain as well. Prochlorperazine (Compazine) can be administered orally (10 mg, three to four times daily), intravenously or intramuscularly (10 mg, three to four times daily), or rectally (25 mg up to twice daily). The promethazine (Phenergan) dose is 25 mg orally, rectally, intravenously, or intramuscularly every four to six hours. Trimethobenzamide (Tigan) is given orally (300 mg, three to four times daily) or intramuscularly (200 mg, three to four times daily). Metoclopramide (Reglan) is available in oral and injectable forms (10 mg orally, intramuscularly or intravenously, every four to six hours). Phenothiazine antiemetics and metoclopramide can cause sedation and occasionally akathisia and tardive dyskinesia. Diphenhydramine (Benadryl) can counteract these neurological side effects.

Serotonin receptor antagonists are highly effective for nausea but probably not as effective for headache as are phenothiazines. However, they do not cause tardive dyskinesia and akathisia. This group includes ondansetron (Zofran, 8 mg orally or intravenously) and granisetron (Kytril, 2 mg orally and 1 mg intravenously twice daily), as well as dolasetron (Anzemet, 100 mg orally and 12.5 mg intravenously) and palonosetron (Aloxi, 0.25 mg intravenously). Aprepitant (Emend) is a neurokinin-1 receptor antagonist, and it is available only orally in 40, 80, and 125 mg tablets and is given once a day.

Corticosteroids

A single dose of dexamethasone (Decadron) (8 mg) or prednisone (60 to 100 mg) can abort a migraine attack that is refractory to triptans and other abortive agents. A tapering six-day course of methylprednisolone (Medrol) is usually reserved for very prolonged (often menstrual) migraines or for the management of medication overuse headaches. The use of corticosteroids has to be limited to a few days a month in order to avoid long-term side effects of these drugs. In cluster headaches, the course of prednisone begins with 100 mg and the dose is tapered off over a period of 10 days. Common side effects of corticosteroids, which can occur even after a single dose, include stomach pain, nausea, mild agitation with insomnia, and more serious side effects.

Ergots

Ergots alone (Ergostat, sublingual) and with caffeine (Cafergot suppositories, Wigraine, tablets) can be quite effective. However, their use has dwindled with the introduction of triptans because they often worsen or cause nausea and other side effects. Suppositories provide rapid onset of action and can be taken even in the presence of severe nausea and vomiting. Reducing the dose of ergotamine/caffeine suppositories to one-quarter or one-half can avoid worsening of nausea and provide effective and rapid relief. The best approach is to have the patient try the suppository between attacks, starting with one-quarter and adding one-quarter every 15 minutes to determine the subnauseating dose. Then this dose can be used during migraine attacks without the fear of causing severe vomiting. If nausea is unavoidable, pretreatment with metoclopramide or prochlorperazine can be tried. The maximum daily dose is two suppositories a day and on not more than two days a week, with the exception of menstrual attacks, where it can be given daily for four to five days, and cluster headaches, when it may be needed for weeks at a time. Ergots are contraindicated in patients with uncontrolled hypertension; cardiac, cerebral, or peripheral ischemia; multiple risk factors for coronary artery disease; and pregnancy.

Dihydroergotamine is very effective for abortive treatment of migraines. This ergot derivative can be given subcutaneously, intramuscularly, intravenously (DHE-45), and intranasally (Migranal). By the time this book is published, an inhaled formulation of dihydroergotamine (Levadex) may be approved by the FDA for the abortive treatment of migraine attacks. While injections of dihydroergotamine can cause or worsen nausea, surprisingly, the inhaled form of this drug rarely does. Pulmonary delivery provides fast onset of action, comparable to the injection. This product may not only be an excellent alternative to injectable sumatriptan, but may also reduce hospitalizations for intravenous dihydroergotamine injections for refractory migraines. It should also work well for the abortive therapy of cluster headaches.

In injectable form a dose of 1 mg of dihydroergotamine is sufficient for most patients, but some may require 2 or 3 mg. The starting dose should be 0.5 mg, repeated in 15 minutes if necessary. Once the total effective dose is established, which could range from 0.5 to 2 mg, that amount can be given for all future attacks. Dihydroergotamine is an effective agent for refractory migraine and can be given to a hospitalized patient intravenously every eight hours for several days. Some patients can avoid hospitalization by self-injecting this medication subcutaneously, although the intravenous route seems to be more effective. Dihydroergotamine can cause or worsen nausea and the injection of an antiemetic, such as prochlorperazine (Compazine) or metoclopramide (Reglan), is often needed.

Opioid Analgesics

Although the use of short-acting opioids to abort acute headaches can be effective, alternative strategies, such as NSAIDs or triptans, are preferred. This is because of a concern about opioid-related side effects, such as nausea and sedation, and the need for the skills and time required to monitor drug-related behavior and thereby ensure and document responsible drug use. There also is an acknowledged stigma associated with opioids, which may lead to reluctance in offering these drugs to patients with severe headache. Nonetheless, parenteral opioids, such as morphine and meperidine (Demerol), continue to be popular in some emergency departments, and some patients in the ambulatory setting respond better to treatment with an oral opioid than other medications used for acute headache. Butorphanol nasal spray (Stadol NS) is the only opioid analgesic approved specifically for the treatment of migraine headaches. Although it is an agonist-antagonist opioid, and therefore less attractive to those with the disease of addiction, abuse can occur and long-term use still requires careful monitoring of both pharmacological outcomes and drug-related behavior. Oral formulations, including popular drugs containing acetaminophen, aspirin, or ibuprofen combined with codeine (e.g., Tylenol #2, #3, and #4), tramadol (e.g., Ultracet), hydrocodone (e.g., Vicodin, Vicodin ES, Vicoprofen), or oxycodone (e.g., Percocet, Percodan), also are commonly tried when headaches are severe and other abortive therapies are ineffective or contraindicated. Opioid formulations often are used during pregnancy because opioids are perceived relatively safe in pregnancy, although they belong in Category C, just like triptans and are probably more deleterious to the fetus than triptans.

Rebound headache has been linked to frequent doses of short-acting opioids, and although the etiologic link between opioid mechanisms and rebound has not been adequately elucidated, it is prudent to consider this risk if patients are using more than two doses per week to abort an acute headache.

Combinations and Miscellaneous Drugs

Combinations of acetaminophen or aspirin with caffeine and a short-acting barbiturate, butalbital (Fiorinal, Fioricet, Esgic, Medigesic), remain stubbornly popular despite complete lack of studies or approval for migraine headaches. Butalbital is banned in Germany and several other European countries because it has limited utility and can cause addiction and dependence.

A limit of 15 to 20 tablets a month is placed on combination drugs or strong analgesics. If a patient takes more than that amount, the medication may begin to worsen the headache through a rebound mechanism. Such patients require prophylactic treatment. The addition of codeine to some of the combinations (Fiorinal with codeine and Fioricet with codeine) improves their efficacy for severe headaches but may result in increased nausea and increased risk for addiction.

Neuroleptics, such as chlorpromazine (Thorazine) and haloperidol (Haldol), can be useful in agitated patients or in those whose nausea does not respond to other medications.

Histamine infusions have been reported by S. Diamond to relieve refractory cluster headaches in 48 of 59 patients hospitalized for this condition. [8]

Parenteral Agents

Migraine patients who fail to respond to oral agents, or because of severe nausea and vomiting cannot take them, often require parenteral therapies. Sumatriptan injections can be easily self-administered by the patient and can be very effective. If sumatriptan injection is ineffective, several other parenteral drugs can be given in doctor's office or an emergency department (see Table 5.2).

Prophylactic Agents

Setting realistic expectations results in improved compliance and ultimately better outcomes. Patients should know potential common side effects of each prophylactic drug they try. They should also know that to avoid side effects, most drugs require slow titration of the dose and that each drug trial may take one to three months. Patients suffering from comorbid depression or anxiety

Table 5.2 Parenteral medications for acute therapy of migraine (excluding opioid drugs)

Drug	Dose	Route/Comments
Dexamethasone (Decadron)	6 to 10 mg	IV push/IM
Dihydroergotamine (DHE-45)	1 mg	SC, IM, IV/often requires coadministration of an antiemetic
Droperidol (Inapsine)	2.5 to 5 mg	IV push/sedating, akathisiais common
Ketorolac (Toradol)	30 to 60 mg	IV push/IM
Magnesium sulfate	1 to 2 g	IV slow 5-min push
Sumatriptan (Imitrex, Sumavel, Alsuma)	4 to 6 mg	SC
Valproate sodium (Depacon)	500 mg	IV push
Antiemetic drugs		
Chlorpromazine (Thorazine)	25 mg IM	Very sedating
Hydroxyzine (Vistaril)	50 to 100 mg	IM
Metoclopramide (Reglan)	10 mg	IV push/IM/nonsedating
Ondansetron (Zofran)	8 to16 mg	IV push/IM/nonsedating
Prochlorperazine (Compazine)	10 mg	IV push/IM

All drugs given by IV push can also be dripped in slowly.

should be offered an antidepressant, while obese patients should be given the option of taking topiramate (Topamax), which has the potential to lower their weight. Patients who are obese or are struggling to maintain normal weight should not be given tricyclic antidepressants or divalproex sodium (Depakote), drugs that can cause weight gain. Hypertension, even if mild, is a good reason to start a patient on a β-blocker or an angiotensin-converting enzyme (ACE) receptor blocker (ARB).

Antihypertensive Drugs

Propranolol (Inderal, Inderal LA), timolol (Blocadren), and other β-blockers are effective prophylactic drugs for migraines. The effective dose for propranolol can be as low as 40 mg daily, but it is usually 80 to 240 mg. Atenolol (Tenormin, 25 to 100 mg) is the least expensive β-blocker and can be taken once a day. Contraindications for the use of β-blockers include bronchial asthma, sinus bradycardia, greater than first-degree cardiac block, congestive heart failure, and diabetes. β-Blockers are often poorly tolerated by young women with low blood pressure. They may also interfere with aerobic exercise, which is one of the most effective nonpharmacological approaches to the treatment of head-aches. Nebivolol (Bystolic) is a β-blocker which appears to be as effective as other β-blockers but with fewer side effects.[9]

Calcium channel blockers are sometimes effective for migraines but are much more likely to benefit patients with cluster headaches. Verapamil (Calan,

Calan SR, Isoptin SR, Verelan) is the most commonly used drug, but it is often not given in a high enough dose. In cluster headache patients, the intensity of pain requires rapid escalation of the dose. Treatment should start with 240 mg of the long-acting formulation and the dose increased every four to five days by 240 mg. It is not uncommon to need 720 to 960 mg (and even higher doses) to control cluster headaches. Common side effects are dizziness, constipation, and ankle edema. It is prudent to perform an electrocardiogram before starting verapamil and after each dose increase.[10] Diltiazem (Cardizem) and nifedipine (Procardia) are similarly only modestly effective for the prevention of migraine headaches. Flunarizine (Sibelium), 5 to 10 mg, is a calcium channel blocker approved for the prevention of migraines in some European countries and Canada, but it is not available in the United States. It is not likely to become available in the United States because of several significant side effects, such as sedation, weight gain, depression, and extrapyramidal (parkinsonian) symptoms.

The ACE inhibitor lisinopril (Prinivil, Zestril), 10 mg, has been reported to be effective in one controlled study in Norway.[11] This double-blind crossover trial of 60 patients showed that lisinopril is effective in the prevention of migraines. Some of the same Norvegian physicians also performed a double-blind crossover trial of an ARB candesartan (Atacand), also in 60 patients.[12] Similarly, candesartan prevented migraine headaches at a dosage of 16 mg daily significantly better than placebo. Olmesartan (Benicar) belongs to this category of drugs and is also presumed to be effective at a dose of 20 to 40 mg daily. While significantly more expensive than β-blockers, they offer a better side effect profile. ACE inhibitors and receptor blockers are contraindicated in pregnant women.

Antiepileptic Drugs

Divalproex sodium (Depakote ER) can effectively relieve migraine headaches. Most migraine patients respond to a daily dose of 500 mg, but some need 1,000 mg or more. Blood levels of this medication can be measured and are useful when escalating the dose beyond 1,000 mg daily. Potential side effects include nausea, indigestion, diarrhea, tremor, hair loss, drowsiness, weight gain, and fatigue. Low platelet counts and liver dysfunction are also possible. This drug is teratogenic (pregnancy Category D), and women of childbearing potential should not take this medication unless other treatments have failed and only if they use a reliable method of contraception.

Topiramate (Topamax) works well for the prevention of both episodic and chronic migraine and is available in 15 mg capsules and 25, 50, 100, and 200 mg tablets. In episodic migraine trials, half of the patients who were given topiramate obtained relief without unacceptable side effects. This is a very popular drug because it causes weight loss in a significant percentage of patients. A patient who is overweight is an ideal candidate for topiramate. However, it has a number of side effects that can be intolerable. Impairment of memory and concentration is the main reason for discontinuing topiramate. Other side effects include perversion of taste (carbonated beverages often have an unpleasant taste), stomach upset, fatigue, anorexia, dizziness, and acroparesthe-sias. Patients should be warned about all common side effects, but particularly acroparesthesias, because this can frighten patients into thinking that they have developed some serious illness. Acroparesthesias tend to subside with time and rarely lead to discontinuation of the drug. Topiramate can cause metabolic acidosis, which can lead to fatigue and other symptoms. When mild, acidosis can be treated with sodium bicarbonate. Drinking sufficient amounts of fluids may help prevent a rare (less than 1%) occurrence of kidney stones. According to the initial clinical trials, kidney stones were thought to occur in less than 1% of patients; however, a more recent study discovered dramatically higher numbers. In this study, researchers evaluated clinically and by CAT scan 75 patients who were taking on average 300 mg of topiramate (the usual effective dose for migraine prophylaxis is 100 to 200 mg) for an average of four years. Symptomatic kidney stones were found in 10.7% and asymptomatic, in 20% of patients.[13] Acute angle closure glaucoma is probably also more common than initially estimated. Topiramate is started at 25 mg with a weekly increase by 25 mg to an average dose of 100 to 200 mg, which can be taken in a single dose, usually at night. Patients sensitive to medication side effects can be started on 15 mg dose with a slower escalation. Some patients require and tolerate doses as high as 800 to 1,000 mg daily. In doses exceeding 200 mg, topiramate begins to interfere with the efficacy of oral contraceptives.

Gabapentin (Neurontin, Horizant, Gralise) is widely used for a variety of conditions because it is the most benign anticonvulsant drug. The dosage forms of the immediate release formulation include 100, 300, and 400 mg tablets and capsules, as well as 600 and 800 mg tablets, while extended release prepara-tion contain 300 and 600 mg. It has been shown to be modestly effective for the prevention of episodic and chronic migraine headaches. It may also help some patients with chronic tension-type headaches. The usual starting dose is 300 mg twice daily with escalation of the dose to 2,400 mg daily and up to 4,800 mg, if the patient reports incremental improvement and if no side effects occur. Potential side effects include dizziness, somnolence, and gastrointestinal symptoms. Gabapentin does not have any significant interactions with other medications.

Little data exist on the use of lamotrigine (Lamictal), pregabalin (Lyrica), levetiracetam (Keppra), and other epilepsy drugs for the treatment of migraine headaches, but these drugs are often tried in patients who fail trials of other, potentially more effective medications. Both gabapentin and pregabalin are approved for the treatment of neuropathic pain.

Antidepressants

Tricyclic antidepressants (TCAs) have been shown to be effective for a va-riety of pain syndromes and for the prevention of migraine and tension-type headaches. Pharmacological treatment of severe persistent headaches begins with nortriptyline (Pamelor) or another TCA. Among TCAs, amitriptyline

(Elavil) has been studied most extensively, but nortriptyline (Pamelor), imipramine (Tofranil), and desipramine (Norpramine) are effective as well and may have fewer anticholinergic side effects. Protriptyline (Vivactil) is the least sedating TCA. If one TCA is ineffective or produces unacceptable side effects, another one should be tried. The starting dose for most TCAs is 10 or 25 mg. The average effective dose, however, is 50 to 75 mg taken once daily in the evening. The exception is protriptyline, which is given in the morning and at an average dose of 10 to 30 mg. TCA serum levels should be checked when there is no or only partial response with no side effects at doses beyond 100 mg (or 30 mg of protriptyline). It helps to explain to patients the antidepressant nature of these medications and that they are used for chronic painful conditions, even in the absence of depression. Otherwise, patients may think that their complaints were interpreted as purely depressive symptoms and they may become resentful and may not return. Possible side effects that patients should be warned about include dryness of mouth, weight gain, drowsiness, and constipation. Urinary retention can occur in men with an enlarged prostate. Some of the contraindications for use of TCAs include concomitant use of MAO inhibitors, recent myocardial infarction, cardiac arrhythmias, glaucoma, and urinary retention. An electrocardiogram should be obtained before the initiation of treatment in children, elderly patients and in those with heart disease.

Antidepressants of serotonin-norepinephrine reuptake inhibitor (SNRI) type have been found to have analgesic and antimigraine properties. Venlafaxin (Effexor, Effexor-XR), desvenlafaxine (Pristiq), and duloxetine (Cymbalta) belong to this group and, unlike TCAs, are less likely to cause weight gain. They do have their own set of common side effects, including insomnia, dizziness, nausea, and sexual dysfunction, and are at times difficult to taper off because of withdrawal symptoms. The dual mechanism of action is responsible for the analgesic properties; however, venlafaxine begins to exhibit this dual mechanism only at a 150 mg daily dose (after a two-week titration, starting with 37.5 mg). Duloxetine exhibits dual mechanism of action at the lowest dose of 20 mg, but the effective dose is achieved by gradual titration to 60 to 120 mg daily. The dose of desvenlafaxine is 50 to 100 mg a day.

Selective serotonin reuptake inhibitors (SSRIs), such as fluoxetine (Prozac, 20 to 80 mg), sertraline (Zoloft, 25 to 200 mg), citalopram (Celexa, 10 to 60 mg), escitalopram (Lexapro, 10 to 20 mg), and paroxetine (Paxil, Paxil CR, 12.5 to 60 mg), do not work for migraines but can be effective for tension-type headaches with fewer side effects than TCAs. These drugs lack the analgesic effect of TCAs, but may help indirectly by reducing anxiety and depression. SSRIs in general do not have potential for weight gain but can cause sexual dysfunction—most commonly, loss of libido or anorgasmia.

Combining SSRIs or SNRIs with triptans can potentially cause serotonin syndrome—a very rare but potentially dangerous drug interaction. Among the symptoms of serotonin syndrome are sweating, tremulousness, diarrhea, tachycardia, hypertension, and hyperthermia. This syndrome has recently received increased attention; however, it remains an extremely rare complication as millions of patients have taken these antidepressants and triptans at the same time without any untoward effects.

Mirtazapine (Remeron, 15 to 45 mg nightly) is a tetracyclic antidepressant similar in its clinical profile to TCAs. It is effective for the prevention of migraine and tension-type headaches, but it also has the similar potential side effects of sedation and weight gain.

MAO inhibitors, such as phenelzine (Nardil, 15 mg three times daily), tranylcypromine (Parnate, 10 mg, 2 to 3 times daily), or selegiline patch (Emsam) are rarely used because of their potential for serious food and drug interactions. Hypertensive crisis can occur from interaction with sympathomimetic and serotoninergic drugs and foods containing tyramine. However, a small number of migraine patients who fail to respond to a variety of other prophylactic medications have a dramatic improvement on MAO inhibitors. These drugs should be tried only in refractory patients. Some of the other potential side effects of MAO inhibitors include sedation, dizziness, weight gain, sexual dysfunction, and constipation.

Lithium (Escalith, Lithobid) is an effective drug for cluster and hypnic headaches. The usual dosage is 600 to 1200 mg daily. Potential side effects include nausea, diarrhea, thirst, insomnia, dizziness, hand tremor, weight gain or loss, rash, constipation, and, after long-term use, diabetes insipidus and hypothyroidism.

Miscellaneous Agents

Tizanidine (Zanaflex) and baclofen (Lioresal) are two muscle relaxants that have been used in the treatment of both chronic migraine[14] and chronic tension-type headaches, particularly when spasm of neck muscles is present. These are very sedating drugs and often can be taken only at night, which is useful for patients with insomnia or those whose headaches tend to start upon awakening or wake the patient from sleep. The usual starting dose of tizanidine is 2 to 4 mg nightly with a slow escalation to 4 to 8 mg three times daily and up to a maximum dose of 12 mg three times daily, which few patients tolerate. Baclofen is started at 10 mg nightly with an increase to 20 mg three times daily and higher, if tolerated.

The Physicians' Health Study showed modest prophylactic effect of aspirin, 325 mg taken every other day,[15] as did the British Doctors Trial, where the dose of aspirin was 500 mg daily.[16] Both studies included only male subjects. A similar study in women that used 100 mg of aspirin daily did not show significant improvement.[17] Naproxen sodium, 1,100 mg daily, and tolfenamic acid (not available in the United States), 300 mg daily, have been shown to prevent migraine attacks in more than one controlled trial. Indomethacin is the drug of choice for the prevention of chronic and episodic paroxysmal hemicrania and hemicrania continua, which appear to be related to cluster headaches. In fact, a complete response to indomethacin is one of the diagnostic criteria for both paroxysmal hemicrania and hemicrania continua. The effective dose of indomethacin for these conditions ranges from 75 to 225 mg daily. Potential gastrointestinal side effects is the major limiting factor in the use of indomethacin, and most patients on daily indomethacin may require gastric protection agents such as proton-pump inhibitors or H2 blockers.

Memantine (Namenda) is an NMDA receptor blocker which is approved for the treatment of Alzheimer's disease. This receptor is involved in a wide variety of physiological processes and is operational in traumatic and ischemic brain injury, as well as pain propagation and cascade of events leading to migraine. Magnesium is another NMDA receptor blocker, although the effect on this receptor may not be the only or the main mechanism of action of magnesium in migraine. Memantine has not been subjected to controlled trials, but several published case series and the author's experience suggest that it may be effective for the prevention of migraines headaches.[18] Memantine has the advantage of a relatively benign side effect propfile. The dose effective for headaches often exceeds that used for Alzheimer's disease. The starting dose is 5 mg daily with escalation to 10 mg twice a day for Alzheimer's disease, and up to 20 mg twice a day for migraines. Anecdotally, combining memantine with magnesium may further improve its efficacy.

The long-term use of corticosteroids has many well-known side effects, and is usually reserved for patients with biopsy-proved temporal (giant-cell) arteritis.

J. Brandes used an atypical antspychotic quetiapine (Seroquel) in a group of refractory migraine patients.[19] Treatment was started with 25 mg and gradually increased to an average dose of 75 mg, and the highest dose of 150 mg daily. Of the 24 migraineurs, 21 had significant improvement in migraine frequency or severity or both, and 18 had reduced disability as measured by MIDAS score. One patient discontinued because of sedation. The atypical antipsychotic drugs have a much lower risk of extrapyramidal side effects and QT segment prolongation compared with phenothiazine drugs. However, these drugs have other potentially serious side effects and should be used sparingly.

Long-term opioid therapy using a long-acting drug (which theoretically reduces concern about rebound or medication overuse headaches) continues to be controversial in headache management, as it is in the management of other types of chronic pain. Nonetheless, pain specialists now agree that a small, carefully selected subpopulation of patients with chronic pain can attain prolonged benefit from these drugs without the development of tolerance, intolerable side effects, or problematic drug-related behavior consistent with abuse or addiction. Clinicians need skills in opioid pharmacotherapy and in risk management to select patients, stratify risk, structure therapy, and monitor outcomes (including analgesia, side effects, function, and drug-related behaviors) over time. A trial of long-term opioid therapy for prophylaxis generally is not considered until a variety of alternative treatments have proven to be ineffective. If a clinician assesses a patient as a potential candidate but lacks the requisite skills in opioid pharmacotherapy and risk management, referral to a specialist with this background may provide the consultative assistance necessary to offer a trial of this approach. In the absence of definitive research on the long-term effectiveness of opioid drugs, these trials are empirical and require careful monitoring and good documentation in the medical record.

It is usually more effective to use the highest tolerable dose of a single drug than to combine smaller doses of two drugs. However, in patients who do not respond to a single prophylactic agent or who obtain only partial relief, a combination of two drugs with different mechanisms of action may be beneficial. Such combinations may include an antidepressant and an anticonvulsant or an antidepressant and a β-blocker. Combining a long-acting NSAID, such as meloxicam (Mobic), with magnesium theoretically may result in improved efficacy and fewer gastrointestinal side effects due to the buffering effect of magnesium.

References

1. Lipton RB, Goldstein J, Baggish JS, et al. Aspirin is efficacious for the treatment of acute migraine. *Headache.* 2005;45:283–292.

2. Kirthi V, Derry S, Moore RA, McQuay HJ. Aspirin with or without an antiemetic for acute migraine headaches in adults. *Cochrane Database of Systematic Reviews* 2010, Issue 4. Art. No.: CD008041.

3. Ferrari M, Roon K, Lipton R, Goadsby P. Oral triptans (serotonin 5-HT$_{1B/1D}$ agonists) in acute migraine treatment: A meta-analysis of 53 trials. *Lancet.* 2001;358:1668–1675.

4. Smith T, Blumenthal H, Diamond M, et al. Sumatriptan/naproxen sodium for migraine: Efficacy, health related quality of life, and satisfaction outcomes. *Headache.* 2007;47:683–692.

5. Bigal ME, Serrano D, Buse D, Scher A, Stewart WF, Lipton RB. Acute migraine medications and evolution from episodic to chronic migraine: a longitudinal population-based study. *Headache.* 2008;48:1157–1168.

6. Wammes-van der Heijden EA, Rahimtoola H, Leufkens HG, et al. Risk of ischemic complications related to the intensity of triptan and ergotamine use. *Neurology.* 2006;67(7):1128–1134.

7. Silberstein SD, Elkind AH, Schreiber C, Keywood C. A randomized trial of frovatriptan for the intermittent prevention of menstrual migraine. *Neurology.* 2004;63:261–269.

8. Diamond S, Freitag FG, Prager J, Gandhi S. Treatment of intractable cluster. *Headache.* 1986;26:42–46.

9. Schellenberg R, Lichtenthal A, Wöhling H, Graf C, Brixius K. Nebivolol and metoprolol for treating migraine: An advance on β-blocker treatment? *Headache.* 2008;48:118–125.

10. Cohen AS, Matharu MS, Goadsby PJ. Electrocardiographic abnormalities in patients with cluster headache on verapamil therapy. *Neurology.* 2007; 69:668–675.

11. Schrader H, Stovner LJ, Helde G, et al. Prophylactic treatment of migraine with angiotensin converting enzyme inhibitor (lisinopril): randomised, placebo controlled, crossover study. *BMJ* 2001;322:19.

12. Tronvik E, Stovne LJ, Helde G, Sand T, Bovim G. Prophylactic treatment of migraine with an angiotensin II receptor blocker: A randomized controlled trial. *JAMA*. 2003;289:65–69.

13. Maalouf NM, Langston JP, Van Ness PC, Moe OW, Sakhaee K. Nephrolithiasis in topiramate users. *Urol Res*. 2011 Aug;39(4):303–307.

14. Saper JR, Lake AE, Cantrell DT, Winner PK White JR. Chronic daily headache prophylaxis with tizanidine: A double-blind, placebo-controlled, multicenter outcome study. *Headache*. 2002;42:470–482.

15. Buring JE, Peto R, Hennekens CH. Low-dose aspirin for migraine prophylaxis. *JAMA*. 1990;264:1711–1713.

16. Peto R, Gray R, Collins R, et al. Randomised trial of prophylactic daily aspirin in British male doctors. *BMJ*. 1988;296:313–316.

17. Benseñor IM, Cook NR, Lee IM, Chown MJ, Hennekens CH, Buring JE. Low-dose aspirin for migraine prophylaxis in women. *Cephalalgia. 2001;21:167–168.*

18. Bigal M, Rapoport A, Sheftell F, Tepper D Tepper S. Memantine in the preventive treatment of refractory migraine. *Headache*. 2008;48:1337–1342.

19. Brandes JL, Roberson SC, Pearlamn SH. Quetiapine for migraine prophylaxis. *Headache*. 2002;42:450–451.

Chapter 6

Interventional Therapies

Botulinum Toxin

Botulinum toxin (BT) was first approved by the FDA in 1989 for the treatment of blepharospasm and strabismus. Injecting BT around the eyes for blepharospasm led to the observation that it erases wrinkles. The widespread use of it for forehead wrinkles led William Binder to the observation that it may relieve headaches.[1] A healthy amount of skepticism greeted initial reports by this plastic surgeon who first observed this effect. However, Mitchell Brin, a movement disorder specialist, confirmed this in his population of patients who, without expecting it, obtained good relief of their headaches along with the relief of their facial movement disorder.[1] After seeing many highly refractory patients respond only to BT, most headache clinics in the United States have started to use BT.[2]

Over 100 published reports have suggested the efficacy of BT, predominantly used as OnabotulinumtoxinA (Botox) in headache patients. A secondary analysis of a large double-blind, placebo-controlled study has shown that BT is effective in treatment of chronic migraines.[3] Two definitive Phase III studies by the manufacturer of OnabotulinumtoxinA (Botox) with over 700 patients in each study confirmed what is widely observed in clinic and what was strongly suggested by other reports and trials: BT is very effective for chronic migraines.[4] These two studies showed a significant reduction of headache days and improved quality of life in patients treated with BT, compared to placebo after two treatment cycles, given 12 weeks apart.

It is less clear how well BT works for episodic migraines and chronic tension-type headaches. This author's experience suggest good efficacy of OnabotulinumtoxinA in the treatment of frequent episodic headaches as well. Beyond a few positive case reports and the author's experience, very little evidence exists about the effect of BT on cluster headaches and trigeminal neuralgia.

The mechanism of action of BT is becoming more clearly understood. The initial speculation that relief of the spasm of pericranial muscles leads to relief may still hold true, at least in part. However, the author observed that BT relieves pain in the bregmatic area where muscles are absent. Recent animal studies by O. Dolly and his collaborators suggest that BT has an effect on sensory neurons, where it inhibits the release of CGRP, one of the major neurotransmitters involved in migraine pathogenesis.[5] BT appears to block the release of other neurotransmitters as well, and may reduce central nociceptive input from pericranial sensory nerves.

Preliminary evidence suggests that patients with constricting type of pain that is going from the outside in, or pain in the eye, are more likely to respond than are those with exploding pain that is felt going from the inside out.[6]

The administration of BT is a relatively simple procedure that takes as little as 10 minutes. Although BT is injected into 15 to 30 sites (typically the forehead, temples, back of the head, and neck), the use of a 30-gauge needle results in little discomfort from this procedure. Injections are usually given into areas of pain, typically into the frontal, temporal, and occipital areas. Some patients benefit from injections into the muscles of the neck, as well as the trapezius and masseter muscles. Studies have shown that with repeated injections, which are usually performed every 3 months, patients obtain better relief with each subsequent treatment. The FDA-approved injection protocol calls for a standard pattern of 31 injections with 155 units of OnabotulinumtoxinA, the protocol that was used in the two largest trials (see Figure 6.1). This author's experience suggests that some patients may benefit from additional injections into masseter and other upper back muscles. Some patients may obtain excellent benefit with 100 units, while a small number of other requires 200 units. The interval between treatments is also somewhat variable, ranging from 10 weeks to 3 months.

After repeated administration of OnabotulinumtoxinA, less than a fraction of 1% of patients can develop neutralizing antibodies to this BT type and stop responding. Such patients may respond to injections of RimabotulinumtoxinB (Myobloc). Myobloc is not the initial choice of BT because its duration of action is a little shorter, side effects are somewhat more common (due to diffusion of the toxin outside injected areas), and pain of injections is greater. Besides OnabotulinumtoxinA, two other type A BTs are available commercially: AbobotulinumtoxinA (Dysport) and IncobotulinumtoxinA (Xeomin). While the three type A BTs are very similar, they are not interchangeable because they are biological products with slightly different properties. The main reason to use only OnabotulinumtoxinA for the treatment of chronic migraines is malpractice considerations since other BT products are not approved for this indication.

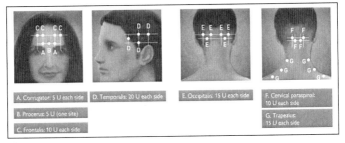

Figure 6.1 OnabotulinumtoxinA (Botox) injection sites for chronic migraine.

The safety of BT has been established in over 20 years of clinical use in millions of patients with various conditions. Among these conditions are torticollis and other dystonias, hyperhydrosis, and spasticity, including that in young children with cerebral palsy who often receive doses much higher than those given to adults with migraines. Side effects, such as bruising, ptosis, weakness of neck muscles, and temporary worsening of head and neck pain, are infrequent (particularly in experienced hands) and mostly mild and reversible, usually within days or weeks.

Nerve Blocks and Trigger Point Injections

Occipital nerve blocks can be effective in aborting a bout of cluster headaches, especially when the nerve is tender on palpation or the patient reports having some pain in the occipital area. These patients also report that pressure in the occipital area provides some relief of orbital pain. Typically, both greater and lesser branches of the occipital nerve are blocked. Similarly, migraine attacks that have an occipital component are likely to be aborted by an occipital nerve block. For migraine, blocking branches of the trigeminal nerve (supraorbital and posterior branch of the mandibular division) can also stop a refractory attack. In the case of cluster headaches and chronic migraines, a mixture of local anesthetic such as lidocaine (Xylocaine) or bupivacaine (Marcaine, Sensorcaine) and a long-acting corticosteroid such as methylprednisolone (Depo-Medrol) or betamethasone (Celestone) is usually used. For abortive therapy of an acute migraine, local anesthetic alone is usually sufficient. The relief of cluster headaches and chronic migraines can last for weeks after a single block.

Injection of a local anesthetic into the trigger points in the neck can provide temporary relief not only of the neck pain, which often accompanies migraine headaches, but also of the headache itself.

It is relatively easy to learn the technique of occipital nerve blocks and trigger point injections. They can provide prompt relief with little risk of side effects.

Patients with migraine and cluster headaches who respond temporarily to the occipital nerve blocks and who do not respond to nondrug approaches, pharmacotherapy, and BT injections are thought to be good candidates for implantation of an occipital nerve stimulator. Subsequent controlled studies have shown that occipital nerve stimulation may relieve migraine headaches regardless of the response to occipital nerve blocks.[5] This therapy is in phase 3 trials and appears quite promising.

Vagus nerve stimulation (VNS) is an approved treatment for refractory epilepsy and depression. Because antiepilepsy drugs and antidepressants are used for the treatment of headaches, this author tried VNS in six patients with chronic highly refractory migraine and cluster headaches.[6] Two out of four patients with migraine and both with cluster headaches had a significant improvement. Other anecdotal observations confirm therapeutic potential of this therapy.[7] This approach is clearly more benign than deep brain stimulation that has been used in refractory cluster headache patients.

References

1. Binder WJ, Blitzer A, Brin MF. Treatment of migraine headaches with botulinum toxin A. *Otolaryngol Head Neck Surg.* 1999;121(no. 2 suppl):162–163.

2. Samton JB, Mauskop A. The treatment of headaches with botulinum toxin. *Exp Rev Neurotherap.* 2006;6:313–322.

3. Dodick DW, Mauskop A, Elkind AH, et al. Botulinum toxin type A for the prophylaxis of chronic daily headache: Subgroup analysis of patients not receiving other prophylactic medications: A randomized double-blind, placebo-controlled study. *Headache.* 2005;45:315–324.

4. Dodick, DW, Turkel CC, DeGryse RE, et al. OnabotulinumtoxinA for Treatment of Chronic Migraine: Pooled Results From the Double-Blind, Randomized, Placebo-Controlled Phases of the PREEMPT Clinical Program. *Headache.* 2010;50:921–936.

5. Meng J, Wang J, Lawrence G, Dolly JO. Synaptobrevin I mediates exocytosis of CGRP from sensory neurons and inhibition by botulinum toxins reflects their anti-nociceptive potential. *J Cell Sci.* 2007;120(16):2864–2874.

6. Jakubowski M, McAllister P, Bajwa Z, Ward T, Smith P, Burstein R. Exploding vs. imploding headache in migraine prophylaxis with botulinum toxin A. *Pain.* 2006;125:286–295.

7. Saper JR, Dodick DW, Silberstein SD, McCarville S, Sun M, Goadsby PJ. Occipital nerve stimulation for the treatment of intractable chronic migraine headache: ONSTIM feasibility study. *Cephalalgia.* 2011;31:271–285.

8. Mauskop A. Vagus nerve stimulation relieves chronic refractory migraine and cluster headaches. *Cephalalgia.* 2005;25:82–86.

9. Klapper J.A., Smith T.R.. Vagus nerve therapy shows potential benefit in patients with migraine and chronic daily headache after 3 to 6 months of treatment. (preliminary results) *Headache.* 2003;43:572.

Chapter 7

Management of Common Conditions

The patient interview is an art that is easy to master, if only one gives the patient a chance to speak. The interview not only is diagnostic, but it can also be therapeutic. Use open-ended questions, such as: "Tell me about your headaches," "Tell me how headaches affect your life," or "What else can you tell me about your headaches?" After presenting the patient with a list of therapeutic options described here, always ask: "What do you think about these options? Do you have any questions about them? And which ones do you want to pursue?"[1]

Establishing the correct diagnosis is not a one-time event but rather an ongoing process. The lack of a biological marker or a test for primary headaches and the reliance on the clinical picture for diagnosis requires constant vigilance and reappraisal, particularly when headaches change in character or worsen in severity or frequency. A migraine sufferer may develop other conditions, such as hypothyroidism, brain tumor, cervicogenic headaches, or magnesium deficiency, which in the beginning may only worsen the typical migraines without any additional signs and symptoms. Typical migraine, tension, or cluster headaches have been reported to occur with the majority of intracranial pathologies, such as vascular abnormalities, tumors, and infections.

After settling on an initial diagnosis, a detailed plan should be discussed and then written out for the patient. Seeing a physician is a stressful event and most people will not remember some important points. A written plan has a better chance of being implemented. It serves as a reminder of things to do and also reassures patients about having many options to control their headaches. A typical plan for a migraine patient may consist of the items detailed in Table 7.1.

It may be easier to have a printed sheet with all of these items, but writing it out by hand for each patient individually will have a stronger impact and make patients somewhat more likely to comply.

It is very useful for a patient to keep a headache diary. The diary helps assess the severity of the problem and, more importantly, gauge the efficacy of treatments undertaken. To improve compliance, the diary should be brief and simple (see Figure 7.1). Instead of a paper diary, patients can use the free Migralex Headache Relief Diary app for iPhone, which was developed by the author. The advantage of this iPhone diary is that it is always with the patient and it allows for recording headache symptoms, treatments, and potential triggers, including automatic recording of barometric pressure, temperature, and humidity at the time of the headache.

Table 7.1 Typical plan for a migraine patient

1 Stop all caffeine, drink sufficient amounts of water, eat regularly, go to bed and wake up at the same time, and get enough sleep.

2 Begin regular aerobic exercise, 30 minutes for three to four days a week.

3 Do one-minute isometric neck exercises 10 times per day.

4 Undergo a course of biofeedback.

5 Take one or more of the following daily: magnesium, 400 mg; CoQ_{10}, 300 mg; feverfew, 100 mg; alpha-lipoic acid, 600 mg; riboflavin, 400 mg; butterbur extract, 150 mg.

6 Consider botulinum toxin injections.

7 Consider prophylactic medications: antidepressants, antihypertensives, anticonvulsants (provide written intake instructions if one is prescribed).

8 For abortive therapy try aspirin/magnesium combination, and if ineffective, take sumatriptan; if sumatriptan is ineffective or if it causes side effects, rizatriptan, or another triptan. If sumatriptan and other triptans are partially effective, combine it with naproxen or aspirin/magnesium combination.

9 Other options: elimination diet, acupuncture, yoga.

If headaches persist, consider sleep study, blood tests, evaluation for temporomandibular joint disorder, cognitive-behavioral therapy.

Date	Pain severity (mild moderate or severe)	Associated symptoms (nausea, vomiting, light and noise sensitivity)	duration (hours)	possible triggers	medication taken	side effects	degree of relief (mild moderate complete)	disability from the attack (mild moderate severe)

Figure 7.1 Headache diary

Migraine

About three-quarters of migraine sufferers report some degree of disability. It is often difficult to assess the impact migraine headaches have on patients' lives. The person sitting in front of you may have a good job, a loving family, and a seemingly normal life, but at the same time be severely disabled. You may be surprised by the difference in your perception and the severe disability scores patients report on MIDAS or HIT-6 scales (Figures 7.2 and 7.3). Both MIDAS and HIT-6 are scientifically valid measures of disability, and help improve communication between patients and physicians. They can also help assess the efficacy of treatment. In addition, it is very useful to have a score on a validated scale when trying to communicate to insurers the degree of patients' disability and their need for expensive treatments such as triptans, topiramate, or botulinum toxin.

Reassurance goes a long way in treating patients with headaches—patients often come with an idea that something is terribly wrong with them, that nothing can be done about their suffering, or that the only thing that can be done is to take drugs that are fraught with dangerous side effects. Detailed history, examination, and, when needed, diagnostic tests will reassure both the physician and the patient about the correct diagnosis. It is important to confirm the biological basis of patients' migraines since, for all of their lives, they have been told directly or have been made to feel that headaches were their own fault or that having headaches was a weakness of character.

Eliminating Triggers

Treatment begins with an attempt to identify triggers and, if possible, to remove them (see Table 7.2).

Many migraine patients are always sensitive to light, develop a migraine from bright light, or cannot tolerate light during an attack. Some of these patients benefit from amber-colored contact lenses or sunglasses.. According to anecdotal reports and some of the author's patients, these lenses allow them to tolerate exposure to sunlight without getting a migraine or reduce the pain of migraine during an attack. Some patients are more bothered by overcast skies more than by sunshine, possibly because of more blue light present, which amber lenses block. Patients who develop headaches from exposure to perfume and other noxious odors can defend themselves by always carrying and, when needed, using Migrastick—a vial of essential oils of peppermint and lavender. Peppermint not only blocks the noxious smells, but has also been shown to have analgesic properties.[2] Migrastick is useful for the relief of milder headaches through its analgesic effect and the massaging action of the roller ball. Keeping a

Table 7.2 **Migraine triggers**
Environmental: loud noise, odors, bright light, heat or cold, high humidity, barometric pressure changes, particulate pollution, carbon monoxide, motion
Nutritional: hunger, dehydration, caffeine, alcohol, aged cheese, chocolate, nuts, citrus fruit, dried food, smoked or pickled food, sulfites, nitrites, MSG, aspartame
Psychological: emotional stress, anxiety, relaxation after stress
Internal: menstrual cycle, pregnancy, menopause, sleep deprivation, too much sleep, sleep disorders, hypothyroidism, magnesium deficiency, dehydration, hunger, physical exertion
Pharmacological: nitrites, drugs for erectile dysfunction, hormonal contraceptives and fertility drugs, antihypertensives, proton pump inhibitors, and many other drugs

Do you suffer from

headaches?

MIDAS QUESTIONNAIRE

INSTRUCTIONS: Please answer the following questions about ALL your headaches you have had over the last three months. Write your answer in the box next to each question. Write zero if you did not do the activity in the last 3 months. Please 'tab' through all five boxes to calculate wour MIDAS score.

1	On how many days in the last 3 months did you miss work or school because of your headaches?	`0` days
2	How many days in the last 3 months was your productivity at work or school reduced by half or more because of your headaches? *(Do not include days you counted in question 1 where you missed work or school)*	`0` days
3	On how many days in the last 3 months did you not do household work because of your headaches?	`0` days
4	How many days in the last 3 months was your productivity in household work reduced by half or more because of your headaches? *(Do not include days you counted in question 3 where you did not do household work)*	`0` days
5	On how many days in the last three months did you miss family, social or leisure activities because of your headaches?	`0` days

Your rating: [＿＿＿＿＿＿＿＿] **TOTAL:** [＿＿] days

A. On how many days in the last 3 months did you have a headache? (If a headache lasted more than 1 day, count each day.)

B. On a scale of 0–10, on average how painful were these headaches? (where 0 = no pain at all and 10 = pain as bad as it can be.)

Scoring

0 to 5, MIDAS Grade I, Little or no disability

6 to 10, MIDAS Grade II, Mild disability

11 to 20, MIDAS Grade III, Moderate disability

21+, MIDAS Grade IV, Severe disability

Figure 7.2 MIDAS questionnaire. Reprinted with permission from Stewart WF, Lipton RB, MD, Dowson AJ, Sawyer J. Development and testing of the Migraine Disability Assessment (MIDAS) Questionnaire to assess headache-related disability. *Neurology* 2001;56:S20-S28; with permission from Lippincott, Williams and Wilkins Publishing.

headache diary can help identify possible food triggers, although many patients become aware of most obvious food triggers without a diary.

Some migraine patients have most of their headaches on weekends. Three possible causes include waking up later than usual and having caffeine withdrawal, too much sleep, and "let-down" after a stressful week. Many migraine patients benefit from a regular sleep schedule, the regular intake of meals, good

HIT-6™

This questionnaire was designed to help you describe and communicate the way you feel and what you cannot do because of headaches.

To complete, please fill in a bubble for each question.

Name: _____ Email Address: _____

1. When you have headaches, how often Is the pain severe?

Never	Rarely	Sometimes	Very Often	Always	
O₁	O₂	O₃	O₄	O₅	HIT6A

2. How often do headaches limit your ability to do usual daily activities including household work, work, school, or social activities?

Never	Rarely	Sometimes	Very Often	Always	
O₁	O₂	O₃	O₄	O₅	HIT6B

3. When you have a headache, how often do you wish you could lie down?

Never	Rarely	Sometimes	Very Often	Always	
O₁	O₂	O₃	O₄	O₅	HIT6C

4. In the past 4 weeks, how often have you felt too tired to do work or daily activities because of your headaches?

Never	Rarely	Sometimes	Very Often	Always	
O₁	O₂	O₃	O₄	O₅	HIT6D

5. In the past 4 weeks, how often have you felt fed up or Irritated because of your headaches?

Never	Rarely	Sometimes	Very Often	Always	
O₁	O₂	O₃	O₄	O₅	HIT6E

6. In the past 4 weeks, how often did headaches limit your ability to concentrate on work or daily activities?

Never	Rarely	Sometimes	Very Often	Always	
O₁	O₂	O₃	O₄	O₅	HIT6F

Figure 7.3 HIT-6TM questionnaire. Reprinted with permission from Quality Metric Inc. © 2008

hydration, and regular cardiovascular exercise. Some migraine sufferers report developing a headache from exercise, and some are unable to engage in any physical exercise. However, most would benefit from regular exercise and could avoid headaches by initially limiting the duration and the intensity of their exercise but engaging in it frequently. Gradually, they will be able to tolerate higher intensity and duration of exercise without developing a headache.

Nondrug Approaches

Many of these methods are not only effective by themselves, but also give patients a sense of control while avoiding potential side effects of drugs.

Even if not completely effective, they may reduce the need for medications. Biofeedback or another form of relaxation training, regular aerobic exercise, isometric neck exercise, acupuncture, dental appliances, massage, magnesium, CoQ_{10}, feverfew, butterbur, alpha lipoic acid, and riboflavin all have some scientific support.

Medications

Acute therapy should be tailored not only to each individual patient, but also to individual attacks. Many patients may respond to a nonsteroidal anti-inflammatory drug (NSAID) when treating milder headaches, and need a triptan or a triptan and an NSAID for severe attacks. Medications, for both acute and prophylactic therapy, should be used at an effective dose. Start all triptans at the maximum recommended dose in most patients, except for those who weigh under 100 pounds (who often report being sensitive to many drugs), or those who have had side effects from another triptan. Many prophylactic medications are titrated up from a low dose, although patients and physicians often fail to escalate the dose high enough, even in the absence of side effects.

Abortive medications are more effective if taken earlier in the attack.[3] Many patients wait to take them in the hope that the headache will not progress, even if it always worsens. Presence of aura allows the patient to take an abortive drug early and sometimes prevent the attack.

Some patients, particularly when prompted, will report that they have premonitory symptoms or prodrome, which can precede the onset of pain by 24 hours. The prodrome can consists of mood changes—depression or elation, yawning or fatigue. Identifying these symptoms may allow some patients to take preventive measures, such as avoiding additional triggers, engaging in relaxation and meditation exercise, or taking asprin with magnesium (Migralex) or naproxen sodium (Aleve), 550 mg twice a day or another abortive drug to prevent the attack.

Comorbidities can help decide on the choice of prophylactic medication (see Table 7.3). Depression, anxiety, and panic attacks are two to three times more common in migraineurs (the relationship is bidirectional), and an antidepressant is an ideal choice for patients with these conditions. Bipolar disorder is also more common in migraine sufferers and, if present, anticonvulsants are

Table 7.3 **Deciding to start prophylactic treatment**
A decision to start prophylactic treatment depends on several factors:
• No response or side effects to abortive agents
• Contraindications for abortive agents
• Comorbid condition (hypertension, depression, anxiety)
• Very frequent attacks
• Patient preference

a good choice. Hypertension is not more common in patients with migraines, but, when present, first try a beta blocker or another antihypertensive drug. In patients with frequent and disabling visual auras, calcium channel blockers and anticonvulsant medications appear to be more effective and B-blockers have been traditionally avoided.

Patients often ask about the duration of prophylactic therapy. Clinical experience suggests that if headaches are very well controlled for a period of six months or so, stopping prophylactic medication may be possible. A large double-blind study of over 800 patients attempted to answer this question.[4] After being on topiramate for 26 weeks, half of the patients were blindly switched to placebo and the other half remained on topiramate for another 26 weeks. The primary outcome measure was number of migraine days in the last four-week period of the first open-label phase compared with the last four weeks of the double-blind phase. There was a statistically significant increase in the number of headache days in patients switched to placebo, although the absolute difference between the placebo and the active groups was only one day. The quality of life as measured by MIDAS was also worse in the placebo group. The authors conclude that benefit continues even if topiramate is stopped after six months of treatment.

Some patients can successfully remain off medication, while others benefit from continued treatment. The impression of many clinicians is that this finding holds true with other prophylactic medications as well.

Chronic Migraine and Medication-Overuse Headaches

The preceding section also applies to chronic migraines. One study found that excessive caffeine consumption is more common in patients with chronic migraine headache.[5] Stopping caffeine leads to actual improvement or improved responsiveness to treatment in the majority of patients. Another study established the link between obesity and the risk of chronic migraines.[6] Reducing weight is much more difficult than stopping caffeine, but it can lead to improvement in headaches. Patients who lose weight by undergoing bariatric surgery also improve.[7] Caffeine, butalbital, and opioid drugs can cause rebound phenomenon and result in medication-overuse headaches. Eliminating caffeine from the diet and stopping caffeine-containing medications can be difficult because of the temporary worsening of pain and associated symptoms. We used to admonish patients to stop all these medications, or else no prophylactic treatment will be effective. Recent studies suggest that topiramate (Topamax) and OnabotulinumtoxinA (Botox) can in fact improve headaches while the patient still takes abortive medications every day.[8,9]

Withdrawal from butalbital-containing medications (Fioricet, Fiorinal, Esgic, Phrenilin, Axotal, Axocet) can be particularly difficult, because in addition to worsening of headaches, patients have symptoms of barbiturate withdrawal. These can include anxiety, irritability, elevated heart and respiration rate, muscle pain, nausea, tremors, hallucinations, confusion, and even seizures. If a patient takes more than four to five tablets containing this drug every day and plans to stop taking them at once, phenobarbital must be given to prevent withdrawal seizures and relieve insomnia (nightly dose of 30 mg if the number of pills is six to eight, 60 mg for withdrawing from eight to ten tablets, and 100 mg if the number is ten to fifteen). Phenobarbital can be discontinued after two weeks with little or no tapering, because its half-life is 96 hours. The rest of the management is similar to that described in the next section on migraine status.

Withdrawal from daily intake of a significant amount (more than about 100 mg of oral morphine equivalent) of short-acting opioid analgesics is done either gradually or by first switching to a long-acting opioid such as methadone, fentanyl patch (Duragesic), or long-acting oxycodone (Oxycontin). Clonidine (Catapres), 0.1 mg, two to three times a day can also relieve some of the withdrawal symptoms, but patients with low blood pressure may not be able to tolerate it. Presence of psychological dependence or addiction requires the involvement of an addiction specialist.

For patients who have developed a medication-overuse headache as a result of overusing opioid drugs, butalbital, or caffeine-containing drugs, replacement of the offending drug with a long-acting NSAID or aspirin/magnesium combination (Migralex) can help break the daily headache cycle. These drugs have not been associated with medication-overuse headache and include diclofenac (Voltaren), meloxicam (Mobic), diflunisal (Dolobid), choline magnesium trisalicylate (Trilisate), nabumetone (Relafen), flurbiprofen (Ansaid), naproxen (Anaprox, Naprosyn), and etodolac (Lodine XL), while regular use of aspirin might even prevent the development of chronic migraines.

Status Migraine and Other Severe Attacks

Treatment of a very prolonged or refractory migraine attack is similar to the approach taken for medication-overuse headache when the overused medication is being stopped. To prepare for the withdrawal of the daily medication (often butalbital, caffeine, and analgesic combination), patients should be given several medications. The patient should be instructed to first try a triptan (orally, intranasally, or subcutaneously), if necessary combined with antinausea medication, given orally or rectally. If headache persists, a single 8 mg dose of dexamethasone (Decadron) and then oxycodone (Percocet, Percodan), 5 to 10 mg can be tried. Very often patients are anxious about stopping medication they have taken for many years and diazepam (Valium, 5 to 10 mg), clonazepam (Klonopin, 0.5 to 1 mg), or alprazolam (Xanax, 0.25 to 0.5 mg) allows them to proceed with the withdrawal and helps them sleep. Giving only a small number of tablets of an opioid analgesic and of a benzodiazepine prevents the risk of developing dependence, tolerance, or addiction to those substances.

Parenteral therapies can be administered not only in the emergency department but also in the office (see chapter 5, Table 5.2). Many emergency departments, with their long waits, harsh lights, noise, and limited choice of medications, are ill suited for treatment of migraine patients. Most of the parenteral drugs can be given in the office by a physician or nurse practitioner without an intravenous line setup but by slow push through a butterfly needle. All of these infusions, with possible exception of ketorolac (Toradol) and dexamethasone (Decadron), should be given with the patient in a recumbent position. One gram of magnesium sulfate in 10 mL of normal saline given over five minutes can abort a severe migraine attack in up to half of migraine patients.[10] Patients should be warned about the warm sensation they will experience during the infusion. If the warmth becomes uncomfortable, the infusion rate is slowed. If magnesium is ineffective within five to 10 minutes of infusion, an intravenous push of 60 mg of ketorolac (Toradol) may abort the attack. If no improvement occurs after another 10 to 15 minutes, an intravenous push of 8 mg of dexamethasone can be given. If nausea is present, 10 mg of metoclopramide (Reglan) is given intravenously. Blocks of the occipital and branches of the trigeminal nerve with a local anesthetic could be tried next. After that, valproate sodium (Depacon) 500 mg can be given intravenously, provided that the pregnancy test in a female patient is negative. One study showed that 2.5 to 5 mg of droperidol intravenously can safely abort a very refractory attack, but potential side effects (prolongation of QT interval, akathisia, sedation) make it the last resort therapy.[11] Because of the relatively high incidence of akathisia, the author administers diphenhydramine (Benadryl) along with droperidol. Both drugs are sedating, and someone has to accompany the patient home.

Several injectable medications can be self-administered by patients or given by a family member. Sumatriptan (Imitrex, Sumavel, Alsuma) is the only drug available in a convenient autoinjector. Some patients may prefer to obtain sumatriptan in vials and use a hypodermic needle, which is less painful than even the needless autoinjector. Using vials also allows patients to titrate the dose, which is particularly useful for patients with frequent attacks of cluster headaches, which may respond to as little as 2 mg. Dihydroergotamine (DHE-45) can be self-administered subcutaneously or intramuscularly, and ketorolac, intramuscularly.

Some patients with very refractory status migraine or who have difficulty withdrawing from butalbital-caffeine combination or another drug require admission to a hospital, daily visits to an infusion center, or daily home visits by a nurse. Dihydroergotamine (DHE-45) given intravenously every eight hours is sometimes called the Raskin protocol after Neil Raskin, who popularized it.[12] Because it can cause or worsen nausea, dihydroergotamine is initially given in a test dose of 0.25 mg, with an additional 0.25 mg given every 10 to 20 minutes to establish an effective subnauseating dose. A typical dose is 1 mg and is given every eight hours. Many patients will require an antiemetic administered before or concurrently with dihydroergotamine. Antiemetics, such as metoclopramide (Reglan) and prochlorperazine (Compazine), reduce not only nausea but also pain. This treatment is usually given for three to five days, despite the official limit of 6 mg of dihydroergotamine per week. In addition to nausea, side effects include muscle cramping, elevation of blood pressure, diarrhea, and chest pressure.

Cluster and Related Headaches

There are three types of treatment for cluster headaches. First, we attempt to abort the entire cluster period with a tapering 10-day course of prednisone, starting with 100 mg a day or with an occipital nerve block. Ambrosini and colleagues showed that suboccipital injection of steroids was better than saline injection in a double-blind study of 10 patients.[13] Intravenous infusion of 1 gram of magnesium sulfate or 500 to 1000 mg of valproate (Depacon) can also abort a cluster period.[14] The second type of treatment is abortive therapy of each individual attack. Sumatriptan (Imitrex) injections, 2 to 6 mg, zolmitriptan nasal spray (Zomig NS), 5 mg, and oxygen are the most effective abortive modalities. Oxygen is administered through a mask (not nasal prongs) at a high flow of 10 L/min, and it usually aborts an attack within 5 minutes. It has no side effects, except for the risk of explosion from open fire (many cluster patients are smokers). Oxygen is practical mostly for patients with strictly nocturnal attacks or for those who stay at home. The third approach, a prophylactic medication, is started if intravenous magnesium, prednisone, or nerve block fails to stop the cluster. The most effective ones include a high dose of verapamil (Calan), divalproex sodium (Depakote), lithium (Lithobid), and topiramate (Topamax). Of these three drugs, topiramate requires the slowest increase of the dose (in order to avoid side effects), although faster escalation than that used for migraine patients can be attempted. Melatonin, 10 mg nightly, has been reported to help some patients and has the advantages of being very benign and inexpensive.[15] In very refractory patients, inpatient treatment with intravenous histamine infusions can be effective. Some cluster patients who have frequent attacks and treat each one with sumatriptan injections can develop a gradual increase in the frequency of attacks, and require sumatriptan injections up to 10 times within 24 hours. These patients may have rebound headaches and require inpatient treatment with intravenous dihydroergotamine, analgesics, or histamine. After hospitalization, they often revert to having one or two attacks a day. A very small number of patients have to continue taking frequent sumatriptan injections for prolonged period of time. The safety of such prolonged therapy is not known, but a recent published report described a 49-year-old woman who failed a wide range of therapies and was taking 12 to 222 mg (in the last year, an average of 150 mg) of injectable sumatriptan daily for a period of 15 years.[16] Since a higher proportion of cluster headache sufferers are smokers and may have other risk factors for coronary artery disease, obtain a stress test prior to initiating treatment with a triptan.

Several studies indicate that some patients with cluster headaches have low testosterone levels. M. Stillman reported that patients with refractory cluster headaches who have low testosterone levels improve when given testosterone replacement.[17]

Paroxysmal hemicranias present with a headache that is similar in description to cluster headaches (except for frequency and duration), but respond dramatically to indomethacin (Indocin) and occasionally other NSAIDs or anticonvulsants. Although rare, hemicrania continua is probably underdiagnosed. It should be considered in patients with constant unilateral headaches even if ipsilateral autonomic features appear only intermittently. A course of indomethacin is diagnostic; patients with hemicrania continua respond dramatically to indomethacin. The drug should be started at 25 mg three times a day and titrated up to 75 mg three times a day before treatment failure is determined. Many patients require gastric protection.

Tension-Type Headaches

Patients with episodic tension-type headaches require little more than over-the-counter analgesics, and they rarely seek medical attention. If someone with what seems like tension-type headache does visit a physician, this fact in itself suggests an underlying pathology that requires thorough investigation. Chronic tension-type headaches do lead patients to seek medical attention, although this is a much less common condition than chronic migraine. Treatment involves all the general measures that are applicable to patients with migraine headaches, with a greater emphasis on biofeedback and cognitive-behavioral therapy. Tricyclic and other antidepressants and, to a lesser extent, botulinum toxin injections can often help. Gabapentin (Neurontin), tizanidine (Zanaflex), and daily administration of an NSAID are other options.

Rhinogenic Headaches

True sinus headaches are usually due to a sinus infection and are accompanied by yellow or green nasal discharge. They are effectively treated with antibiotics and decongestants. Polyps and minor inflammation of sinus walls, seen on computed tomography (CT) scans or magnetic resonance imaging (MRI), do not cause headaches. It is not unusual for chronic sinusitis to worsen someone's migraine headaches, but patients and physicians often misinterpret these as purely sinus-related headaches. Treatment in such patients should be directed not only at the sinuses (surgery is scandalously overused) but at the underlying migraine headaches as well. Enlarged turbinates and deviated septum do not cause headaches with the possible exception of a contact point. Several reports suggest that removing this contact point between the septum and the lateral wall of the nasal passages may improve headaches.[18] A simple test can sometimes predict success of this surgery: If intranasal lidocaine drops provide temporary relief, then surgery has a better chance of relieving headaches.

Cervicogenic Headaches

Elimination of potential contributors, such as cradling the telephone handset and carrying heavy bags on the shoulder, provides relief for many patients. Treatment of these headaches consists of a regimen of isometric (see Figure 7.1) and other neck exercises, which have been shown to be as effective as manual therapy. Typical manual therapy by chiropractors carries a small but significant risk of carotid or vertebral artery dissection and should be discouraged.

However, if high-velocity manipulations are avoided, manual therapy can be beneficial. Sleeping with a soft cervical collar can also help as the collar prevents the patient from assuming awkward positions while asleep. The collar should be narrow and not very restrictive so as not to interfere with sleep. Patients should not wear it during the day because this may cause weakening of neck muscles due to inactivity and lead to worsening of muscle spasm. NSAIDs, tricyclic and SNRI antidepressants, gabapentin, and tizanidine are medications that can help but can be difficult to tolerate by the elderly, who are more likely to be afflicted by these headaches. Biofeedback, acupuncture, occipital nerve blocks, and botulinum toxin injections are safer and often more effective options than medications or can be combined with medications. More invasive procedures, such as epidural steroid injections, percutaneous radiofrequency neurotomy, and facet joint injections, carry a small but not negligible risk of serious complications and should be tried only if other therapies fail. In cases of significant disc disease with a compromised neural foramina and epidural space, surgical intervention may be necessary. However, mild and moderate disc bulges are very common in the general population and do not cause persistent neck pain or headaches.

Benign Exertional Headaches

Exercise can provoke a headache that can range from mild to excruciating and is usually throbbing in quality. The headache can occur at the start of exercise or only with overexertion. When exertional headache occurs for the first time, obtain an urgent CT scan of the brain to evaluate possible subarachnoid hemorrhage. If neck stiffness and other signs of meningeal irritation are present, a lumbar puncture is performed to detect subarachnoid hemorrhage, even when the CT scan is negative. Persistence of these headaches may require MRI to investigate for other abnormalities. Stress test may reveal cardiac ischemia as a possible cause, although headache alone is a very unusual presentation of angina. In the absence of an organic cause, treatment begins with physical conditioning. Encourage patients to begin regular aerobic exercise several times a week, starting with low intensity and brief duration and gradually increasing both intensity and duration. If even mild exertion triggers a headache, aspirin with magnesium (Migralex), ibuprofen (Advil), or naproxen (Aleve) taken prior to exercise may prevent the headache. These medications need to be taken only for the first few weeks, and then the headaches will often stop occurring. In refractory cases, daily intake of indomethacin or a beta blocker can provide relief.

Sex-Induced Headaches

Sexual activity can bring on a headache prior to or at the point of climax. These headaches are much more common in men. The headache can last a few minutes or a few hours, and can be dull or feel like an explosion in the head without associated symptoms. An NSAID taken before sexual activity can prevent this headache. Physical conditioning helps, as do beta blockers. Sex-induced headache in older individuals can be cervicogenic in origin, and changing position during intercourse can eliminate the headache.

Benign Intracranial Hypertension (Pseudotumor Cerebri)

This idiopathic syndrome is characterized by elevation of intracranial pressure with normal composition of the cerebrospinal fluid (CSF) and in the absence of a space-occupying lesion or enlarged ventricles. Conditions that have been associated with pseudotumor cerebri include obesity, hypervitaminosis A, isoretinoin, hypoparathyroidism, pesticide poisoning, head trauma, systemic disease, tetracycline, oral contraceptives, and corticosteroids. Diagnosis is established when elevated CSF pressure, normal MRI (although ventricles tend to be small), and no other underlying illness are present. Swelling of the optic nerve on funduscopic examination is almost always present. Differential diagnosis includes thrombosis of cerebral veins, malignant hypertension, meningoencephalitis, meningitis, optic neuritis, ischemic optic neuropathy, neoplasm of optic nerve, neoplasm of spinal cord, intracranial mass, and Lyme disease. Headache of pseudotumor is usually constant, can be pulsatile, and may be associated with nausea, photophobia, and phonophobia. Blurred vision and visual field defects should raise the alarm and lead to aggressive efforts to lower intracranial pressure in order to prevent permanent loss of vision. Acetazolamide, 250 to 1000 mg daily in two to three divided doses, can provide relief, as can weight loss in obese patients. Topiramate (Topamax), similarly to acetazolamide, seems to be selectively inhibiting carbonic anhydrase in the choroid plexus. Topiramate can also produce weight loss. If medications fail, repeated lumbar punctures can be performed, but in some patients they provide only short-lived relief. Lumboperitoneal shunt is an effective treatment for refractory patients. Patients threatened with visual loss may require optic nerve sheath fenestration. Even in the absence of visual symptoms, visual field testing should be done regularly as long as the headache persists.

Secondary Headaches

Postconcussion headache is very common. There is little correlation between the severity of head injury and the likelihood or the severity of postconcussion headaches. Headache often is only one of many postconcussion symptoms, which can also include poor concentration, dizziness, insomnia, impaired memory, depression, anxiety, and mood fluctuations. Patients who sustain a whiplash injury without a head trauma, often during a car accident, can exhibit similar symptoms. It is likely that sudden acceleration and deceleration causes the same effect on the brain as does a direct impact. Neck muscle spasm could be a contributing factor to these headaches. Secondary gain issues in cases of car accidents or in cases of other compensable accidents make the diagnosis and treatment more difficult.

Treatment needs to address all of the postconcussive symptoms. Cognitive rehabilitation, tricyclic or SNRI antidepressants, anticonvulsants, and the passage of time usually lead to improvement. Acupuncture, biofeedback, magnesium, botulinum toxin injections, and physical therapy directed at the neck can also provide relief.

Headache due to temporomandibular joint (TMJ) disorder is diagnosed by the presence of pain in the TMJ, tenderness of the joint on palpation, limited range of movements, or noise from the joint on movement. Many of these patients clench or grind their teeth at night and often have hypertrophied masseter muscles. Treatment of an acute headache due to TMJ dysfunction consists of soft diet and an NSAID for a period of one to two weeks. Chronic headaches are sometimes treated with a dental appliance that is worn at night or both at night and during the day. In severe cases of joint degeneration, joint replacement becomes necessary. In the absence of structural joint disease or malocclusion, antidepressants, muscle relaxants, and some anticonvulsants, such as gabapentin, can be effective. Botulinum toxin injections into the masseter and temporalis muscles are also very effective.

Post-lumbar puncture headache occurs in about 25% of patients undergoing a spinal tap. The use of thinner or conical spinal needles reduces the incidence of post-lumbar puncture headaches. Contrary to popular belief, bed rest following a lumbar puncture does not prevent these headaches. The headache can be accompanied by neck stiffness, photophobia, nausea, and tinnitus. When a patient does develop a headache, bed rest, hydration, caffeine, and analgesics can provide relief. Most patients improve within a few days. If there is no improvement after two to three days (or sooner if the headache is debilitating), the patient should receive a blood patch. This procedure involves withdrawing 15 to 20 mL of patient's venous blood and injecting it into the epidural space at the same level where the lumbar puncture was performed. This stops the leakage of CSF and relieves the headache, sometimes within minutes of the procedure.

Spontaneous intracranial hypotension is a relatively rare condition caused by leaking of the CSF, and which can occur upon straining or without an obvious trigger. A contrast MRI shows meningeal enhancement. This finding is also seen in post-lumbar puncture headache. Searching for the CSF leak may require CT-myelography. Once the leak is found, an epidural infusion of saline, a blood patch, or surgical repair may be required.

Cerebral vein thrombosis causes headaches in the vast majority of patients. Other presenting signs and symptoms include papilledema, depressed level of consciousness, seizures, and focal neurological deficits due to venous infarctions. About one-quarter of patients present only with a headache. This condition is more common in women after delivery and on oral contraceptives, in patients with cranial infections, and in those in hypercoaguable states. In the majority of patients, headaches resolve with time. The diagnosis is established by MRV, although CT and MRI can show infarctions and brain edema. Treatment includes anticoagulation and, in some cases, diuretics and anticonvulsants.

Ischemic strokes and transient ischemic attacks are accompanied by a headache in 40% of patients, while hemorrhagic strokes almost always present with a headache.

Headache associated with an intracranial neoplasm can present as a typical migraine, tension headache, or even cluster headache. The established perception that brain tumor usually causes a headache upon awakening is not supported by facts. The most common type of headache that occurs upon awakening is migraine.

Meningitis headache also lacks any specific characteristic, but the presence of neck stiffness, fever, and other systemic symptoms makes the diagnosis easier.

Aneurysmal headache usually stems from rupture of the aneurysm, which results in death for 40% of patients before they reach the hospital. In those who survive and are seen by the physician, a typical complaint is that it is the "worst headache of my life." Sentinel headaches that portend a rupture can occur in some patients, and possibly result from minor bleeds from the aneurysm or just stretching of the wall of the aneurysm. These headaches are usually milder and lack distinguishing characteristics.

Headache due to dissection of a vertebral or carotid artery is usually unilateral and is accompanied by neck pain. In severe cases the dissection leads to a stroke, but it can also be a fairly benign condition. It can result from a trivial injury or even vigorous shaking of the head as well as more serious neck injuries, and chiropractic manipulation. The author encountered a 56-year-old woman who developed internal carotid artery dissection as a result of shaking her head after the shower to get water out of her hair, something she has done for years without a problem. The diagnosis is made by MRA. Treatment consists of anticoagulation, although controlled trials to prove its efficacy have not been done.

Hydrocephalus can be of communicating or obstructive type, and both can cause headaches. Obstructive hydrocephalus results from obstruction of CSF flow and is caused by aqueductal stenosis, Chiari malformation, or a neoplasm, or occurs after bacterial infection. Communicating hydrocephalus can result from a head injury or meningitis or without an obvious cause. Shunting of the CSF from the lateral ventricle to the peritoneal cavity usually relieves the hydrocephalus and the headaches.

Typical headaches of Chiari malformation are occipital in location with associated neck pain. When the herniation is severe, coughing can provoke a headache, and neurological signs and symptoms are usually present. The severity of Chiari malformation is determined by the degree of herniation of the brainstem and cerebellar tonsils into the foramen magnum and is measured in millimeters. A herniation of less than 5 mm on MRI, especially if there is ample space around the tonsils, is not likely to cause headaches. Symptomatic Chiari malformation is treated by surgical enlargement of the foramen magnum.

Giant cell or temporal arteritis rarely occurs in people younger than fifty. The headache is typically unilateral and continuous and is accompanied by tenderness over the temporal artery. Some patients have associated polymylagia rheumatica and mild anemia. The diagnosis is established by a characteristic clinical picture, significantly elevated ESR and CRp, but the definitive diagnosis is made by temporal artery biopsy. It is important to be certain about this diagnosis because this condition often condemns the patient to life-long treatment with corticosteroids. Patients may need only 5 mg of prednisone daily, but most cannot completely stop it because of the recurrence of symptoms with a corresponding rise of the CRP levels. These patients require close monitoring for possible long-term side effects of corticosteroids. If left untreated, this condition can lead to strokes and loss of vision.

Headaches that result from epileptic activity are common and usually easy to diagnose. Rarely, patients have headaches that are produced by nocturnal or subclinical seizures. Ambulatory electroencephalographic monitoring is more likely to document epileptic activity than a routine electroencephalogram. It is more common for epilepsy patients to have migraine headaches not related to their seizures. Having one condition makes the patient more likely to have the other, and the relationship is bidirectional.

Medication-induced headaches are extremely common, can occur from almost any drug, and are usually easy to diagnose. However, at times the link between medications such as oral contraceptives, estrogen, proton pump inhibitors, H2 blockers, asthma medications, or antihypertensive drugs and headaches is not obvious and should be considered when most other etiologies are not found. Proton pump inhibitors by reducing gastric acidity can cause vitamin and mineral deficiencies, including vitamin B12 and magnesium, which can worsen headaches after prolonged use.

Hangover (also known as overindulgence headache) is not a common reason patients seek medical attention, but they might inquire about the best treatment, short of abstinence. Dehydration and magnesium depletion (the latter documented in animal and human studies) are presumed causes of this headache and associated symptoms of hangover. Hydration and aspirin/magnesium combination (Migralex) is an effective therapy. Patients should be cautioned not to take aspirin or other NSAIDs while drinking alcohol because of the increased risk of gastric side effects. Acetaminophen should not be consumed with alcohol because of the increased hepatotoxicity.

Neuralgias

Occipital neuralgia is more common in older individuals, although it can occur at any age and may be present in patients who also have migraine headaches. The symptoms include pain in one or both occipital areas with associated numbness and paresthesias. The pain is often worse upon awakening in the morning or after a nap. Dentists who work for long periods of time with their heads tilted, or secretaries and sales personnel who cradle the telephone handset on their shoulder, are more susceptible to this condition. In the elderly, arthritic changes in the cervical spine can cause pain, which in turn can cause muscle spasm and entrapment of the occipital nerve. Examination is notable for numbness or tenderness in the distribution of the occipital nerve, and frequently spasm and tenderness of suboccipital muscles. The most effective and quick-acting treatment is block of the occipital nerve (usually of both the greater and lesser branches) with a local anesthetic, lidocaine (Xylocaine) or bupivacaine (Marcaine), combined with a long-acting corticosteroid such as methylprednisolone (Depo-Medrol) or betamethasone (Celestone). Other approaches include isometric neck exercise (see Figure 4.1), NSAIDs, tricyclic antidepressants, gabapentin, and OnabotulinumtoxinA (Botox) injections. If the symptoms are worse in the morning, a soft cervical collar worn only for sleep can be dramatically effective. The collar needs to be narrow so that it is not too uncomfortable and does not interfere with sleep. The purpose of the collar is to prevent extremes of neck position while asleep, which leads to worsening of muscle spasm and pain upon awakening.

Pathognomonic feature of trigeminal neuralgia is pain in one or more of the branches of the trigeminal nerve that is described as electric shock-like in quality and very brief in duration. Pain that is primarily aching, burning, throbbing, or pressure-like, or that lasts longer than a few seconds, is incompatible with this diagnosis. Some patients do have aching pain between bouts of the excruciating electric shocks. Pain of trigeminal neuralgia never lasts for more than several seconds, although it can occur in a rapid succession for longer periods of time. Many patients develop pain upon touching a certain trigger spot on their face or, more often, on speaking, chewing, while brushing the teeth, or without any provocation. Neurological examination is normal. The underlying cause of this condition, which is more common in the elderly, is compression of the trigeminal nerve by a blood vessel at the point of exit of the nerve from the brainstem. Age-related or hypertension-induced hardening of the blood vessel, usually an artery, causes increasing pressure on the nerve and loss of myelin insulation. This loss of insulation causes cross-talk or short-circuiting in the nerve bundle, which manifests itself by electric-like pain. Treatment begins with carbamazepine (Tegretol) or oxcarbazepine (Trileptal), but other anticonvulsants, such as phenytoin (Dilantin) and the muscle relaxant baclofen (Lioresal), can be effective. Anesthetizing the trigger area can provide short-term relief, while botulinum toxin injections have been reported to provide longer-lasting relief in a handful of reported cases and in the author's experience. Despite modest evidence, Onabotulinumtoxin (Botox) injections may be worth trying because they are extremely safe and the amount required to treat trigeminal neuralgia is relatively inexpensive. Percutaneous radiofrequency ablation of the corresponding portion of the trigeminal ganglion and other similar percutaneous destructive procedures can be effective—although these treatments carry a very small, but very frightening, possibility of causing anesthesia dolorosa. Curative therapy, pioneered by P. Jannetta, consists of occipital craniotomy with trigeminal nerve decompression, which is achieved by placing insulation made of Teflon between the nerve and the compressing blood vessel.[19]

Glossopharyngeal neuralgia is much less common than trigeminal neuralgia. It is usually milder but also causes electric-like pain deep in the ear (tympanic type) or in the tongue and throat (glossopharyngeal type). It is treated with the same medications as trigeminal neuralgia.

References

1. Hahn S. Communication in the care of the headache patient. In Silberstein SD, Lipton RB, Dodick DW, eds. *Wolf's Headache and Other Head Pain*, 8th ed. New York: Oxford University Press; 2008:805–824.

2. Gobel H, Schmidt G, Soyka D. Effect of peppermint and eucalyptus oil preparations on neurophysiological and experimental algesimetric headache parameters. *Cephalagia*. 1994;14:228–234.

3. Cady R, Martin V, Mauskop A, et al. Efficacy of rizatriptan, 10 mg administered early in a migraine attack. *Headache*. 2006;46:914–924.

4. Diener HC, Agosti R, Allais G, et al. Cessation versus continuation of 6-month migraine preventive therapy with topiramate (PROMPT): A randomized, double-blind, placebo-controlled trial. *Lancet Neurol*. 2007;6:1054–1062.

5. Scher AI, Stewart WF, Lipton RB. Caffeine as a risk factor for chronic daily headache: A population-based study. *Neurology*. 2004;63:2022–2027.

6. Bigal ME, Liberman JN, Lipton RB. Obesity and migraine. A population study. *Neurology*. 2006 66:545–550.

7. Bond DS, Vithiananthan S, Nash JM, Thomas JG, Wing RR. Improvement of migraine headaches in severely obese patients after bariatric surgery. *Neurology*. 2011;76(13):1135–1138.

8. Silberstein SD, Lipton RB, Dodick DW, et al. Efficacy and safety of topiramate for the treatment of chronic migraine: A randomized, double-blind, placebo-controlled trial. *Headache*. 2007;47:170–180.

9. Dodick DW, Mauskop A, Elkind AH, DeGryse R, Brin MF, Silberstein SD. Botulinum toxin type A for the prophylaxis of chronic daily headache: Subgroup analysis of patients not receiving other prophylactic medications: A randomized double-blind, placebo-controlled study. *Headache*. 2005;45:315–324.

10. Mauskop A, Altura BT, Cracco RQ, Altura BM. Intravenous magnesium sulfate relieves migraine attacks in patients with low serum ionized magnesium levels: A pilot study. *Clin Sci*. 1995;89:633–636.

11. Silberstein SD, Young WB, Mendizabal JE, Rothrock JF, Alam AS. Acute migraine treatment with droperidol: A randomized, double-blind, placebo-controlled trial. *Neurology*. 2003;60:315–321.

12. Raskin NH: Repetitive intravenous dihydroergotamine as therapy for intractable migraine. *Neurology*. 1986;36:995–007.

13. Ambrosini A, Vandenheede M, Rossi P, et al. Suboccipital injection with a mixture of rapid- and long-acting steroids in cluster headache: A double-blind placebo-controlled study. *Pain*. 2005;118:92–96.

14. Mauskop A, Altura BT, Cracco RQ, Altura BM: Intravenous magnesium sulfate relieves cluster headaches in patients with low serum ionized magnesium levels. *Headache*. 1995;35:597–600.

15. Leone M, D'Amico D, Moschiano F, Fraschini F, Bussone G. Melatonin versus placebo in the prophylaxis of cluster headache: A double-blind pilot study with parallel groups. *Cephalalgia*. 1996;16:494–496.

16. Kallweit U, Sandor PS. Sumatriptan in Excessive Doses Over 15 Years in a Patient With Chronic Cluster Headache. *Headache*. 2011;51:1546-1548.

17. Stillman M. Testosterone replacement therapy for treatment refractory cluster headache. *Headache*. 2006;46:925–933.

18. Behin, F., Behin, B., Bigal, M. and Lipton, R. Surgical treatment of patients with refractory migraine headaches and intranasal contact points. *Cephalalgia*. 2005;25: 439–443.

19. Barker FG, Jannetta PJ, Bissonette DJ, et al. The long-term outcome of microvascular decompression for trigeminal neuralgia. *N Engl J Med*. 1996 334:1077–1084.

Chapter 8

Special Populations

Headaches in Pregnancy and Menstrual Migraines

Migraine headaches stop in two-thirds of pregnant women, especially in the second and third trimester. They also stop after menopause, and at around the same age in men. In pregnancy, all attempts are made to avoid medications by using nonpharmacological therapies such as biofeedback, massage, application of ice, and aromatherapy. Nausea can be treated with motion sickness bands (Sea-Band, BioBands, Psi-Bands), which are wrist bands with a pressure point placed two inches above the wrist crease. This is an acupuncture point and has been proved to relieve nausea induced by motion, pregnancy, chemotherapy, and post surgery.[1] Metoclopramide is in Category B and is safe in pregnancy. When necessary, acetaminophen alone or with an opioid analgesic is tried first. Ibuprofen and naproxen can be used only in the first two trimesters of pregnancy. Triptans are considered to be a safer approach than allowing a woman to have uncontrolled migraine attacks with nausea, vomiting, and dehydration. For prophylactic therapy in pregnancy the author uses magnesium, intravenously or orally, before trying any other intervention. Propranolol, which is in Category C, is considered safe and is often used as the first-line drug, but atenolol is in Category D and is contraindicated. Amitriptyline is generally considered safe, although it is also in Category C. Divalproex sodium and topiramate are in Category D and are contraindicated. OnabotulinumtoxinA (Botox) is in Category C, but since it has a negligible systemic absorption it is probably safer than any prophylactic drugs in the same Category. The author has treated pregnant women with OnabotulinumtoxinA without any adverse outcomes.

Menstrual migraines that are difficult to control with abortive drugs can be treated with mini-prophylaxis: starting a nonsteroidal anti-inflammatory (NSAID) drug such as naproxen, triptans, or beta blockers the day before expected headache. This strategy works only when the period and the attendant headache are highly predictable. Another option for women with menstrual-related migraine is to take an oral contraceptive pill (OCP). Because migraines are often triggered by fluctuations in estrogen, stabilization of estrogen levels with low-dose (35 μg of estrogen or less) monophasic contraceptives can decrease the intensity and duration of headaches in these patients. Estrogen and progestin combinations, such as drospirenone with ethinyl estradiol (Yasmin, Yaz), may also reduce other premenstrual symptoms, such as fluid retention and mood disturbance.

If menstrual headaches persist on this type of contraceptive, continuous contraception may be considered. There are OCPs designed to be taken continuously for three months (Seasonale, Seasonique) or even for a year (Lybrel), although any monophasic OCP can also be used continuously. This strategy is not always effective, because some women break through and still have periods and headaches. Women interested in OCPs as part of their headache treatment should discuss this option with their gynecologist or family doctor. In the author's experience OnabotulinumtoxinA can significantly reduce the severity of pain of menstrual migraines.

Estrogen-containing OCPs are relatively contraindicated in women who have migraine with aura, because they increase the risk of strokes. However, recent data suggests that this risk is dose-related and that newer OCP with lower amounts of estrogen are safer. Patients who have migraine with or without aura should reduce all other modifiable risk factors for stroke such as smoking, high cholesterol, and hypertension. OCPs should be avoided in women with risk factors for cardiovascular disease and any type of migraine.

Headaches in Children

Just as there are not enough neurologists to see even a fraction of all adult migraine sufferers, there are even fewer pediatric neurologists. Pediatricians and family physicians usually treat headaches in children; however, the treatment of an older child is similar to that of an adult, so that an adult neurologist or any other interested physician can undertake it. A detailed history, physical examination, and often a magnetic resonance imaging (MRI) study are necessary to establish the benign nature of the headache. Strong family history of similar headaches may obviate the need for an MRI, but in the majority of children such an imaging study is indicated. Differentiating migraine from tension-type headache is difficult in children, because the headache may be accompanied by only one or two migraine features and the attack usually lasts an hour or two. The default diagnosis, just like in adults, should be migraine. Less common conditions in children are abdominal migraine or cyclical vomiting, where no other migraine symptoms are present and where a thorough search for every other cause of these symptoms needs to be performed before settling on this diagnosis. Cluster headaches are uncommon in children, but this diagnosis should also be kept in mind.

Treatment usually begins with an attempt at elimination of possible triggers such as irregular sleep schedule (which is highly prevalent in teenagers), lack of physical activity, poor diet, excessive caffeine intake, and very often stress. Biofeedback is very effective in children, who often learn this technique much faster than adults. Parental discord and tension in family life or difficult school environment often aggravate migraine headaches. The author has seen many children stop having headaches after going off to a boarding school or college.

Daily supplementation with magnesium oxide, 9 mg/kg, can help prevent migraines in some children, according to study by F. Wang and his colleagues.[2]

Other preventive therapies include TCAs, such as amitriptyline (Elavil, 5 to 10 mg in young children, 10 to 25 mg nightly in older ones; an electrocardiogram is done prior to initiation of treatment to detect conduction defects) and beta blockers, such as propranolol (Inderal, 1 to 2 mg/kg daily in two divided doses). Cyproheptadine (Periactin) is a popular drug for the prevention of migraine in children, but unfortunately it has never been shown to work and usually it does not. OnabotulinumtoxinA (Botox) injections appear to be as effective in children as in adults with frequent or chronic migraines, and the author has used it to treat refractory chronic migraines in children as young as 10 years.

NSAIDs such as ibuprofen or, in children over 12, an aspirin/magnesium combination (Migralex) and naproxen (Aleve) can be very effective. For younger children, liquid formulations or suppositories of NSAIDs or acetaminophen can provide faster relief and are particularly appropriate when nausea or vomiting is present. Brief duration of attacks made it very difficult to do clinical trials of triptans in young children, since after one to two hours, the headache is gone with or without medication. Only two of the seven available triptan are officially approved for children. Rizatriptan (Maxalt) is approved for children 6 and older and almotriptan (Axert) is approved for children older than 12. However, extensive experience with triptans over the past 20 years in children suggests that all these drugs are safe and effective. While in adults the highest available dose formulation should be used, in children the lowest one is started with. However, if a child weighs over 100 pounds, a higher dose may be appropriate from the start. Nasal spray usually provides faster relief. Although zolmitriptan (Zomig NS) is a little more efficacious than sumatriptan (Imitrex NS), the availability of a 5 mg dose of sumatriptan spray makes it the first choice for younger children.

Headaches in the Elderly

A new onset of headaches in an older person is more likely to herald a serious illness such as a metastatic or primary brain tumor, temporal arteritis, glaucoma, or a metabolic disorder such as hypothyroidism. Occipital neuralgia and cervicogenic headaches are common causes of new onset of headaches. Another common trigger of headaches in the elderly is medications. The list of drugs that can cause headaches is extensive, and if a particular medication is not vitally important, it should be stopped or, if possible, replaced by a drug from a different class. Medication-overuse headaches are also common in the elderly and can be successfully treated. Hypnic headache occurs almost exclusively in the elderly.

Migraines often stop after menopause in women but also decline in frequency in men, although not to the same extent—the 3:1 ratio of female to male migraineurs at a younger age becomes 2:1 in the elderly. Treatment of migraine in the elderly is more challenging because the elderly are more likely to have other medical conditions and to take other drugs, which could interfere with migraine medications. The use of triptans is not contraindicated in the elderly, and the author encountered an 85-year-old woman who was taking sumatriptan with excellent relief for over 10 years. However, the elderly are likely to have coronary artery disease, and even asymptomatic and otherwise perfectly healthy patients should undergo at least a nuclear exercise stress test prior to starting a triptan.

The use of prophylactic medications in the elderly should be undertaken with caution because the half-life of many drugs can be longer and therefore upward titration should be slower. The elderly are more sensitive to side effects, and the starting dose of most drugs should be lower.

Poor nutritional status and chronic illness often lead to magnesium and other deficiencies, which can be easily corrected. Patients with frequent headaches who have multiple medical problems and who cannot tolerate drugs may respond well to OnabotulinumtoxinA (Botox) injections. Acupuncture and biofeedback can also be very effective.

The elderly who are depressed are more likely to complain of somatic than affective symptoms. Therefore, a complaint of headache in the absence of another cause should raise the possibility of depression. Treatment with antidepressants such as SSRIs can be very effective and safer than with TCAs, albeit the latter ones are more effective analgesics.

Headaches in Patients with Comorbid Conditions

Psychiatric Disorders

While headache can be the main somatic symptom of depression in the elderly, in most migraine sufferers, depression is a separate condition. The risk of falling into depression is about three times higher in a patient with migraines, but risk of developing migraines is also three times higher in someone who is depressed, suggesting a shared underlying pathophysiology rather than causative link.[3] Depression occurs in 80% of patients with chronic migraine. The prevalence of other psychiatric conditions, such as anxiety, panic attacks, bipolar disorder, and obsessive-compulsive disorder, is also much higher in migraine sufferers. Chronic pain sufferers, including those with headaches, are more likely to have been abused physically, emotionally, or sexually. Some of these patients suffer from post-traumatic stress disorder. There are many effective screening tools that can detect these conditions when symptoms are not obvious and the physician's time is short. In case of depression, incorporating just two questions into the initial visit forms that patients complete will diagnose depression in 90% of patients:

1. Have you been bothered a lot in the last month by feeling sad, down or depressed?
2. Have you been bothered a lot in the last month by loss of interest or pleasure in your daily activities?

Treatment of headaches without addressing psychiatric comorbidity is more difficult, and probably less successful. Fortunately, treatment of headaches, anxiety, and depression often can be accomplished with the same drug: a TCA or a SNRI antidepressant. The use of cognitive-behavioral therapy can also provide relief for both conditions. It is very helpful to involve a mental health provider early in the treatment.

Fibromyalgia

Migraine is more common in patients with fibromyalgia, which is characterized by widespread pain, fatigue, memory difficulties, and sleep disorders.[4] Patients with fibromyalgia appear to have a wind-up of certain brain neurons and sensitization of the nervous system. Functional brain MRI studies show that pain processes are augmented in patients with fibromyalgia compared to controls. The therapies for fibromyalgia—TCAs, SNRIs such as duloxetine (Cymbalta), pregabalin (Lyrica), and gabapentin (Neurontin)—along with physical therapy can also provide effective relief for migraines.

Irritable Bowel Syndrome

Irritable bowel syndrome (IBS) is characterized by cramping, abdominal pain, bloating, constipation, and diarrhea. It occurs in up to 20% of the population. Migraine sufferers have a higher incidence of IBS, and patients with IBS are more likely to suffer from migraine headaches, as well as from fibromyalgia and depression.[5] IBS is treated with diet, probiotics, medications, and stress management. In patients with predominance of diarrhea, treatment with a TCA can address most of the symptoms. Diarrhea can lead to malabsorption of magnesium, cyanocobalamine, and other vitamins. Oral magnesium supplementation can contribute to diarrhea and in such patients, an intravenous infusion of magnesium sulfate can be very effective without causing any side effects. Vitamins B_2, $B_{12,}$ D, and CoQ10 may also be depleted, and supplementation can improve patients' headaches and other symptoms.

Sleep Disorders

Sleep disorders are more common in patients with chronic than with episodic headaches. Some of the sleep disorders associated with headaches include obstructive sleep apnea, periodic limb movement disorder, restless leg syndrome (RLS), and insomnia. Insomnia appears to be a risk factor for tension-type headaches. In addition to morning headaches, symptoms of sleep apnea may include snoring, nonrefreshing sleep, gastroesophageal reflux, and erectile dysfunction. Headache patients need to be screened for sleep disorders as treatment of obstructive sleep apnea, RLS, and insomnia seems to improve headaches.[6] It is important to take into account the fact that insomnia is also comorbid with depression. Cluster headache patients have a high incidence of sleep apnea, and interestingly, one of the abortive therapies for cluster headaches is inhalation of pure oxygen, although treating sleep apnea has not been proved to relieve cluster headaches.

The mnemonic *REST* is useful in identifying a sleep disorder: the *restorative* quality of sleep, *excessive* daytime somnolence or fatigue, the presence of *snoring*, and sufficient *total* sleep time.

Treatment of insomnia usually begins with sleep hygiene, elimination of caffeine, relaxation exercises, and self-hypnosis, but it can also include the use of hypnotic drugs. Obstructive sleep apnea is treated with weight loss, elimination of smoking and alcohol consumption, dental appliances, soft palate surgery, and continuous positive airway pressure.

References

1. Ezzo J, Streitberger K, Schneider A. Cochrane Systematic Reviews examine P6 acupuncture-point stimulation for nausea and vomiting. *J Altern Complement Med.* 2006;12:489–495.

2. Wang F, Van Den Eeden SK, Ackerson LM, et al. Oral magnesium oxide prophylaxis of frequent migraine headache in children: a randomized, double-blind, placebo-controlled trial. *Headache.* 2003;43:601–610.

3. Jette N, Patten S, Williams J, Becker W, Wiebe S. Comorbidity of migraine and psychiatric disorders—A national population-based study. *Headache.* 2008;48:501–516.

4. Ifergane G, Buskila D, Simiseshvely N, Zeev K, Cohen H. Prevalence of fibromyalgia syndrome in migraine patients. *Cephalalgia.* 2006;26:451–456.

5. Tietjen GE, Herial NA, Hardgrove J, Utley C, White L. Migraine comorbidity constellations. *Headache.* 2007;47:857–865.

6. Rains JC, Poceta JS. Headache and sleep disorders: Review and clinical implications for headache management. *Headache.* 2006;46:1344–1341.

Chapter 9

Typical Cases

A "Plain" Migraine

Abigail was a 32-year-old woman who had suffered from severe headaches for the past 15 years. Her headaches were unilateral, severe in intensity, and pulsatile, with photophobia and phonophobia but not nausea, and they were made worse by light physical activity. She did not have any aura symptoms. They occurred two or three times a month, and each attack lasted three days. Typical triggers were work-related stress, weather, and her menstrual cycle. She had tried sumatriptan (Imitrex), 100 mg, eletriptan (Relpax) 40 mg, and zolmitriptan (Zomig) 5 mg, with no relief. Review of organ systems revealed anxiety, insomnia, some depression, coldness of extremities, and premenstrual syndrome. She did not use tobacco and did not consume alcohol or caffeine. She was single and worked full-time. Her mother suffered from migraine headaches. Physical examination was normal. Her body mass index was 25. The MIDAS score was 12.

Assessment: Intractable Migraine Headaches without Aura and with Moderate Level of Disability; Comorbid Anxiety and Depression

Initial Plan

1. Regular aerobic exercise.
2. Biofeedback and cognitive therapy.
3. Magnesium and CoQ_{10} supplements.
4. Venlafaxine, 37.5 mg daily with a gradual increase to 150 mg or higher, if needed.
5. For abortive therapy, rizatriptan (Maxalt), 10 mg was prescribed.

On her return visit one month later, Abigail reported having her usual three migraines, but they were milder and responded well to rizatriptan. She also noticed a mild improvement in her mood on 150 mg of venlafaxine.

During the second month of treatment, she had only one menstrual attack and it was relieved by rizatriptan. After three months of treatment, her MIDAS score dropped to five and she could abort most of her attacks with magnesium/aspirin (Migralex) and only rarely needed rizatriptan.

Take-Home Messages

1. If one triptan is ineffective or causes side effects, another one may work well without side effects.

2. Do not prescribe drugs with a potential for weight gain, such as tricyclic antidepressants or divalproex sodium (Depakote), to young women who are already overweight or are struggling to maintain a normal weight. Depakote is teratogenic—another reason to avoid it in fertile women.
3. Do not feel that you should be scientific and try only one treatment at a time, because you will likely lose the patient before you can help her. Combine medications with nonpharmacological approaches.

"Complicated" Migraine

Brittany was a 27-year-old woman who was referred by a neurologist for possible nonpharmacological therapies. She had suffered from headaches for the past five years. The headaches were unilateral, severe in intensity, pulsatile, and associated with rapid onset of nausea, as well as photophobia and phonophobia. The pain was made worse by light physical activity. These attacks would occur twice a month, with one attack taking place the day before her period. The patient also reported that in the previous two years, she had four episodes of loss of vision on the left side of her visual field, followed by slurred speech, numbness, some clumsiness, and mild weakness of the left arm. This entire sequence of symptoms lasted 30 to 45 minutes and was followed by a headache that was more severe than usual. Her neurologist obtained a magnetic resonance image of her brain, gave her the diagnosis of complicated migraine, and informed the patient that triptans were contraindicated. Hydrocodone with acetaminophen, butalbital/caffeine/acetaminophen, and naproxen were ineffective.

Her family history was negative for headaches. She did not smoke or drink alcohol, but she drank three to four cups of coffee every day. Her physical examination was normal.

Assessment: Migraine with Typical Aura
Initial Plan

1. Reduce caffeine intake (from none, to no more than one small cup of coffee daily).
2. Start regular aerobic exercise.
3. Take a supplement of magnesium, CoQ_{10}, riboflavin, and feverfew.
4. Zolmitriptan nasal spray was prescribed for abortive therapy of her attacks.

Two months later, Brittany's headache frequency was reduced to one attack per month, and these were aborted by zolmitriptan within 30 minutes and without any side effects.

Take-Home Messages

1. Hemiplegic migraine is very rarely seen, even at a headache clinic.
2. The presence of mild subjective weakness is common in patients who also report numbness, and it does not indicate the diagnosis of hemiplegic migraine.

3. Even if true hemiplegic migraine is present, an experienced neurologist may prescribe a triptan. A series of case reports has been published in which patients with hemiplegic migraine were safely given triptans. However, because vascular complications do, albeit very rarely, occur and because of the attendant legal risks, try to avoid using triptans as the first or second approach to abortive therapy and think of prophylaxis sooner than you would otherwise do. Another reason for more aggressive prophylaxis is the disability and anxiety of anticipating and suffering from hemiplegic attacks.

Too Old for Migraines

Charles was a 75-year-old man who developed daily headaches two weeks prior to his visit. The headaches started in the left temporal area but then spread to the right side as well. The headache was severe and woke him from sleep. It was not accompanied by nausea, but he did have some photophobia and phonophobia, as well as worsening with light physical activity. He never suffered from headaches in the past. His primary care physician obtained a series of blood tests, all of which were normal. Erythrocyte sedimentation rate (ESR) was 11.

A chiropractor obtained an x-ray of his cervical spine and discovered degenerative changes with some subluxation of C_3 on C_4. A series of neck adjustments did not relieve his headaches. An oral surgeon was consulted, but no cause of headaches was found.

To relieve the pain, Charles had been taking Tylenol, up to eight tablets daily, with minimal relief. A butalbital/aspirin/caffeine combination was also ineffective.

His medical history included repair of an abdominal aortic aneurysm as well as a coronary artery stent placement several years earlier. He also had bouts of depression in the past, but not recently.

Review of organ systems was negative for malaise, fever, joints, or muscle pains.

His examination was normal, without tenderness of the temporal arteries, but his temporomandibular joints were somewhat tender on palpation.

MRI and MRA scans of the brain were completely normal. CRP level was 3.6 (normal <0.8 mg/dL), while his second ESR was 80.

Assessment: Presumed Temporal Arteritis

Prednisone, 60 mg daily, was started for presumed temporal arteritis and a temporal artery biopsy was scheduled for the next day.

A temporal artery biopsy revealed an active lympho-histiocytic infiltration, scattered giant cells, and intimal fibrosis, findings consistent with temporal arteritis.

Charles' headache improved significantly within two days of initiating prednisone, 60 mg daily.

Take-Home Messages

1. Migraines do not begin in people who are in their sixties or seventies.
2. Normal ESR is not unusual in patients with temporal arteritis; obtain a CRP and repeat the ESR. CRP is not only more sensitive than ESR in detecting temporal arteritis, but ESR results can be easily affected by improper handling of the specimen.
3. Start prednisone only if you are certain that a biopsy will be performed within a few days. Do not commit an elderly person to life-long prednisone treatment without a biopsy confirmation since this carries a high risk of serious side effects.

A Man Who Banged His Head Against the Wall

Dillon was 37 and had been suffering from severe headaches for three years. He had bouts of headaches every spring and fall, and they would last about two months. Similar headaches also occurred throughout the year, but only once or twice a month. His headaches occurred at night, when they woke him from sleep, but he also had attacks during the day. On some days he had up to three or four attacks. The pain was very intense, lasting 30 to 40 minutes, and was always localized to the right eye. It was accompanied by nasal congestion and clear discharge from the right nostril. His right eye became teary, conjunctiva injected, and the right eyelid drooped slightly during the attack. He did not have sensitivity to light or noise. The patient would become very restless and agitated and paced the floor; when the pain became very intense, usually five to 10 minutes after the onset, he would hit the right side of his head with his fist and even hit his head against the wall. Hitting his head provided momentary relief.

Dillon attributed his headaches to allergies and sinus problems and had seen an allergist and two otolaryngologists. CT and MRI of his brain, allergy testing, and routine blood tests were normal. He was treated with antibiotics for presumed sinus infections, allergy medications, and decongestants, all with little relief. He gave up smoking a year after his headaches began, without any improvement. His mother suffered from migraine headaches. His physical examination was normal.

Assessment: Episodic Cluster Headaches

Cluster headaches were diagnosed, and the patient was given a 10-day tapering course of prednisone, starting with 100 mg. This aborted his attacks, but they returned when the dose of prednisone was reduced to 30 mg daily. He was started on extended release formulation of verapamil, 240 mg daily, with a dose increase by 240 mg every five days to 960 mg, which resulted in cessation of attacks. An electrocardiogram was obtained before initiating verapamil and before each increase of dosage. Dillon was also prescribed injectable sumatriptan, which provided excellent relief of individual attacks. In the beginning, before verapamil became effective, he needed up to three injections a day.

Take-Home Messages

1. Cluster headaches can occur outside cluster periods.
2. Proper trial of prednisone requires a starting dose of 100 mg.
3. Verapamil is effective for the prophylactic treatment of cluster headaches, but sometimes only at a high dose. As long as constipation, ankle edema or other side effects do not become a problem, the dose can be increased even beyond 960 mg.
4. Electrocardiogram should be done after each dose increase to monitor for possible cardiac side effects.
5. Sumatriptan has a very short half-life and is safe to administer more often than the approved two-a-day limit.

Pregnant with Headache

Eloise was a 29-year-old woman who had been suffering from migraine headaches since puberty. For the past year she had a very stressful job, which worsened her migraine frequency to once or twice a week. They were more severe premenstrually. Each attack lasted a full day. The attacks were severe, with associated nausea, vomiting, photophobia, and phonophobia. She had no relief from acetaminophen, ibuprofen, naproxen, and butalbital, but responded to sumatriptan (Imitrex) and was able to go to work; however, she was still not completely symptom-free. Her MIDAS score of 26 indicated severe disability. The patient did not abuse caffeine, exercised regularly, and had no other obvious migraine triggers. She had a strong family history of migraines. Her physical examination was normal. Eloise had just gotten married and was thinking of trying to conceive. She was concerned about taking rizatriptan or any other medications. A course of biofeedback was recommended, but she had little free time and her insurance would not cover it. Magnesium oxide, 400 mg, and 300 mg daily of CoQ_{10} were started. Because of the safety record of opioid drugs in pregnancy, for abortive therapy she was prescribed acetaminophen with codeine, but it caused worsening of nausea with little relief of pain. After one month on supplements the headache frequency dropped from about six attacks per month to three or four, but the severity did not improve. She still had to take sumatriptan, 100 mg, once or twice for each attack. After discussing potential risks and benefits, she decided to continue taking sumatriptan even after getting pregnant. Within two months of getting pregnant, her headaches completely stopped and did not recur until two months after delivery. She had a normal pregnancy and delivered a healthy boy. Six months after delivery, her headaches returned. While breastfeeding, she was advised to take sumatriptan and discard the milk obtained within six hours after taking it.

Take-Home Messages

1. Migraines improve during pregnancy (and menopause) in two thirds of women, presumably due to lack of estrogen fluctuations.

2. Magnesium and CoQ_{10} should be tried in all patients.
3. Triptans are relatively safe in pregnancy based on the data from pregnancy registries, which contain data on more than 1,000 women.
4. If preventive therapy is needed for frequent migraine attacks during pregnancy, botulinum toxin, beta blockers, and tricyclic antidepressants can be used, although they are all category C.

"Sinus" Headache

Fiona was 34 years old and had suffered from headaches for most of her adult life. The headaches had always been frontal and perinasal in location and were accompanied by some nasal congestion with small amounts of clear discharge. The pain was usually throbbing and the patient would experience sensitivity to light and noise, but never had nausea. Headaches lasted up to three days. Her headaches had some seasonal patterns—more common in the fall and spring, but she never had more than a week or two without headaches. She had seen several allergists and ENT specialists and had sinus surgery on two occasions in an attempt to cure her headaches. Only once or twice a year, she would have a sinus infection with colored nasal discharge, which would resolve with antibiotics. Despite normal CAT and MRI scans, Fiona was convinced that she had sinus headaches and was referred to the headache clinic by her next ENT specialist who felt that her sinuses were healthy. She had been taking large amounts of ibuprofen (up to 2400 mg a day) with limited relief, but it allowed her to function, albeit with severe disability, judging by the MIDAS score of 32. The patient consumed three or four tall cups of Starbucks coffee every day. Review of her organ systems was remarkable for anxiety and insomnia. Medical history was otherwise unremarkable. Family history was positive for similar sinus headaches in her father. Fiona had stayed home to care for her two young children. Her physical examination was normal.

Assessment: Migraine without Aura

The diagnosis of migraine without aura was established. All coffee and ibuprofen were stopped, with initial worsening of her headaches for three days. The attacks were successfully treated with rizatriptan (Maxalt), 10 mg three times a day as needed. She also started regular aerobic exercise and a magnesium supplement. Within three months, her headache frequency dropped to two or three a month, and these were controlled by rizatriptan. Her disability level improved to mild with the MIDAS score of eight. Her sleep improved and anxiety subsided.

Take-Home Messages

1. Sinus symptoms, except for colored nasal discharged, are common in patients with migraine headaches.
2. Seasonal fluctuations in headache frequency are common in migraine sufferers.

3. A Starbucks tall-sized coffee contains 280 mg of caffeine—twice the amount of most other brands and triple the amount of a regular-sized cup of coffee.
4. Caffeine is one of the worst offenders in causing rebound headaches.

A Headache that Would Not Go Away

Ginny was a 42-year-old woman who had been suffering from headaches since puberty. The frequency of attacks began to worsen in her late twenties, and by the age of 30 she was having daily headaches. Her headaches, if left untreated, would become severe, pulsatile, with sharp pains in one eye, and were accompanied by nausea, vomiting, photophobia, and phonophobia. The patient had seen several neurologists and tried approximately 20 different prophylactic medications including B-blockers, calcium channel blockers, tricyclic antidepressants, anticonvulsants, muscle relaxants, CoQ_{10}, magnesium, and riboflavin, all with no relief. She had been getting relief from all triptans and was taking them daily. Ginny alternated between sumatriptan, zolmitriptan, and eletriptan because they were equally effective and caused no side effects, but she could only get a limited amount of each from her insurance company. Once she stopped taking triptans for two weeks because they were thought to be causing rebound headaches, but her headaches did not improve. Because of triptans, she was able to hold a job as a high school teacher, although her disability score was 22, in the severe range—she missed many weekend activities and had occasional severe attacks when she ran out of triptans. She was married and had two teenaged children. Ginny did not drink any caffeine. Her family history was positive for headaches in her maternal grandmother. Physical examination was normal.

Assessment: Chronic Migraine

The diagnosis of chronic migraine was made and botulinum toxin injections were performed. After three successive treatments with botulinum toxin three months apart, her headache frequency gradually decreased and the disability score dropped to ten. She continued to take six to eight tablets of zolmitriptan a month.

Take-Home Messages

1. Headaches can occur daily for many years.
2. Taking triptans daily is not an optimal treatment, but allows some patients to live productive lives and does not appear to cause any long-term side effects.
3. Rebound headaches from triptans happen but are rare.
4. Botulinum toxin sometimes works when no other treatment does.

"Hormonal" Headache

Hermione was a 39-year old woman who, for the previous five years, had been having only one headache each month; however, this headache, which started the day before her period, lasted for a total of three days. During these three days, the patient was incapacitated by the headache because of unremitting pain, nausea, and vomiting. Other symptoms included frequent leg muscle cramps and coldness of extremities, both of which worsened during her periods. Sumatriptan injections and prochlorperazine suppositories would provide partial relief, but would not restore her to normal functioning because of the residual pain, fatigue, and drowsiness. Opioid analgesics relieved the pain, but also sedated her. She was given propranolol to take daily, but at 60 mg she developed dizziness without relief of her headaches. Topiramate caused cognitive impairment. Continuous contraception stopped her periods for only two months and then her period broke through and was accompanied by a severe migraine. Dexamethasone, 8 mg daily for the three days of headache, provided sufficient relief to allow her to go to work, but she still had a mild headache and nausea and could function at about 50% of her capacity. Oral magnesium supplementation did not help, but an injection of 1 g of magnesium sulfate during an attack produced dramatic relief without any side effects. Hermione tried increasing her oral supplementation with magnesium oxide from 400 mg to 800 mg, but developed diarrhea. Trials of chelated and slow release forms of magnesium did not cause diarrhea but also did not prevent her menstrual migraine. The patient went on to receive monthly premenstrual infusions of 1 g of magnesium sulfate with complete prevention of her migraine attacks. When she traveled and was unable to receive her infusion, the severe headache returned.

Assessment: Menstrual Migraine with Magnesium Deficiency

Menstrual and non-menstrual migraines may not respond to triptans and other drugs if magnesium deficiency is present and is not corrected. Sometime magnesium provides only partial relief, but it will often also improve response to abortive drugs.

Take-Home Messages

1. Leg muscle cramps and coldness of extremities (or feeling cold in general) are symptoms suggestive of magnesium deficiency.
2. Oral magnesium supplements can be poorly absorbed (genetic factors are postulated).
3. Menstrual migraine attacks can be very difficult to treat despite epidemiological studies suggesting that on average they are no more refractory than nonmenstrual attacks.
4. Intravenous infusions of 1 g of magnesium sulfate are extremely safe and can be easily administered through a slow, five-minute push.

"Nothing Ever Worked for Me"

Irene was a 49-year-old woman who had been having daily headaches for more than 15 years. Her headaches were present continuously and involved her entire head with a throbbing quality of pain and daily episodes of nausea, but not photophobia or phonophobia. She had tried B-blockers, TCAs, and several anticonvulsants, all with little relief. Botulinum toxin injections provided some relief and improved her functioning, although the level of disability remained severe: 65 on the MIDAS scale. Triptans were ineffective for abortive therapy, and she was taking six tablets of butalbital/acetaminophen/caffeine combination daily. The patient reported that "this is the only medicine that works for me." The reason for her visit was that her primary care physician was reluctant to prescribe 180 tablets monthly. An MRI of her brain and a battery of blood tests were normal.

Review of organ systems revealed anxiety, insomnia, constipation and neck pains. Her family history was positive for migraine headaches in her mother and 23-year-old daughter. Irene was married and did not work. The patient did not drink any alcohol or caffeine and did not smoke. Her neurological examination was normal, except for spasm and tenderness of her neck muscles.

Assessment: Medication-Overuse Headache

Diagnosis of medication-overuse headaches was made, and a treatment plan was proposed to the patient. Despite her pronounced anxiety about stopping her medication, she was willing to try to stop it. She was told to stop the drug at once and was prescribed a tapering course of prednisone, starting with 80 mg daily with daily reduction of the dose by 10 mg. She was also given prescriptions for 30 mg of phenobarbital, to be taken nightly for two weeks to prevent withdrawal seizures; prochlorperazine suppositories, 25 mg, to be taken as needed for nausea; and 30 tablets of diazepam, 5 mg, to be taken every six hours as needed for anxiety. She was also prescribed dihydroergotamine nasal spray to be taken as needed for her headaches. The patient was started on magnesium oxide, 400 mg and butterbur, 150 mg and was urged to start regular aerobic exercise. Irene was able to stop her butalbital-containing medication and her headache frequency decreased to one or two attacks a week. These attacks responded to dihydroergotamine nasal spray, but because of nasal irritation she was switched to oral sumatriptan, which did not help in the past, but was very effective after detoxification. Her anxiety and insomnia also lifted.

Take-Home Messages

1. Patients who do not respond to multiple treatments need to be evaluated for medication overuse as well as possible underlying metabolic or structural lesion.
2. Butalbital and caffeine-containing drugs can cause refractory headaches, anxiety, insomnia, and physical and psychological dependence.
3. Stopping butalbital abruptly can cause a withdrawal seizure, which needs to be prevented by phenobarbital, 30 to 100 mg a day.

4. Other withdrawal symptoms need to be managed aggressively to ensure successful detoxification.
5. Triptans become effective when the overused drug is stopped.

"Numb" Headache

Jonathan, a 59-year-old executive, was very concerned about his headaches, which began after a long airplane ride two weeks before his visit. The pain was constant and mostly involved the right side of his forehead. He also felt numbness and a pins-and-needles sensation over the right occipital area. He was afraid that this was a sign of an impending stroke and was eager to have an MRI of his brain. He denied having nausea, photophobia, phonophobia, or any other neurological symptoms, but did admit to having some neck discomfort. Jonathan did not try any medications because he did not like to take any and because he did not want to mask his symptoms. He was in good health, exercised regularly, did not abuse alcohol, and drank only one cup of coffee daily. Jonathan had had a normal annual evaluation by his internist three months earlier. His physical examination was normal, except for diminished sensation over the right occipital area and tenderness of suboccipital muscles.

Assessment: Occipital Neuralgia

Jonathan seemed to accept the diagnosis of occipital neuralgia caused by muscle spasm triggered by sleeping in an awkward position on the airplane. An MRI was going to be obtained if he did not improve within two weeks. He was offered a choice of conservative therapy, which would include sleeping with a soft cervical collar, isometric neck exercise, and an anti-inflammatory drug or doing a nerve block. He chose the nerve block. Both the greater and the lesser occipital nerves on the right side were blocked with 2 mL of 1% lidocaine and 20 mg of methylprednisolone acetate suspension (Depo-Medrol). Jonathan had complete relief of his headache, which did not recur.

Take-Home Messages

1. Frontal headache can originate in the occipital area.
2. Occipital neuralgia often does not produce pain typical of most other neuralgias—it is not electric-like or lancinating, but dull and achy, and is often accompanied by paresthesias.
3. An occipital nerve block is a simple and very useful procedure for occipital neuralgia, as well as cluster and migraine headaches.

Index

Page numbers followed by t indicate a table

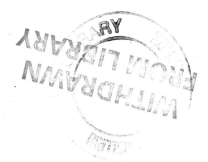